PRAISE FOR THE

'A heart-wrenching exploration of the struggle for autonomy amidst dwindling resources, *The Merge* perfectly captures a modern world obsessed with controversial solutions for problems it has created... I was riveted from the first page to the last.'
Ling Ling Huang, author of *Immaculate Conception*

'Chilling, claustrophobic and deeply unsettling, *The Merge* is a brilliant, unforgettable exploration of memory, control and freedom.'
Carole Hailey, bestselling author of *The Silence Project*

'A disturbing, heartbreaking and gripping read, which manages to explore capitalism, technology, personal identity, climate change, human rights and over-population without ever losing sight of its central characters and their vividly drawn lives.'
Jo Harkin, author of *Tell Me an Ending*

'Grace Walker creates an uncanny world so rich and all-encompassing that it's hard to believe it's not real... it's clear that Walker poured her all into this future classic of the genre.'
Jodie Matthews, author of *Meet Me at the Surface*

'An arresting, deeply imaginative debut. *The Merge* is both a gripping speculative drama and a moving meditation on memory, family and control. Grace Walker also asks what we're willing to surrender for those we love and her questions linger long after the final page.'
Freya Bromley, author of *The Tidal Year*

'With *The Merge*, Grace Walker takes a clever speculative premise, and creates a dystopian world that feels frighteningly plausible; filled with compelling characters struggling to come to terms with the new reality. Terrifying and fascinating.'

                                          Guy Morpuss, author of *Five Minds*

'I read *The Merge* in one frenzied weekend… Walker has a frighteningly good imagination, but the most frightening thing of all is that the world she's created doesn't feel all that outlandish… This is a story that will stay with me. Timely, important, and beautifully written.'

                                      Silvia Saunders, author of *Homesick*

THE MERGE

Grace Walker

MAGPIE
BOOKS

A Magpie Book

First published in the United Kingdom, Republic of Ireland and Australia
by Magpie Books, an imprint of Oneworld Publications Ltd, 2025

Copyright © Grace Walker, 2025

The moral right of Grace Walker to be identified as the
Author of this work has been asserted by her in accordance
with the Copyright, Designs and Patents Act 1988

All rights reserved
Copyright under Berne Convention
A CIP record for this title is available from the British Library

ISBN 978-1-83643-049-0
eISBN 978-1-83643-051-3

Printed and bound in Great Britain by Clays Ltd, Elcograf S.p.A.

This book is a work of fiction. Names, characters, businesses, organisations, places and events are either the product of the author's imagination or are used fictitiously. Any resemblance to actual persons, living or dead, events or locales is entirely coincidental.

Quotation from *The Cocktail Party* by T.S. Eliot. © 1950 by T.S. Eliot.
Used by permission of Faber and Faber Ltd.

No part of this publication may be reproduced, stored in
a retrieval system, or transmitted, in any form or by any means,
electronic, mechanical, photocopying, recording or otherwise,
or used in any manner for the purpose of training artificial intelligence
technologies or systems, without the prior permission of the publishers.

The authorised representative in the EEA is eucomply OÜ,
Pärnu mnt 139b–14, 11317 Tallinn, Estonia
(email: hello@eucompliancepartner.com / phone: +33757690241)

Oneworld Publications Ltd
10 Bloomsbury Street
London WC1B 3SR
England

Stay up to date with the latest books,
special offers, and exclusive content from
Oneworld with our newsletter

Sign up on our website
oneworld-publications.com

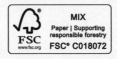

For Gary and Jim.

What is hell? Hell is oneself.
Hell is alone, the other figures in it
Merely projections. There is nothing to escape from
And nothing to escape to. One is always alone.

T.S. Eliot, *The Cocktail Party*

They warned us about the grief.

They explained how, when the day came, it would feel as though someone were dying. They reassured us that grieving was normal, to be expected. There was a whole week of sessions dedicated to it.

I watched the speakers during the grief sessions, studying them as they told us about their own experiences. I wasn't fully listening, catching the odd word, the occasional consoling phrase. I was too busy trying to catch them out, waiting for something to slip and give them away.

Nothing happened, obviously. The speakers were flawless in their delivery. I should have accepted that. I should have given up and paid attention to what they were saying.

If I'd properly listened at the sessions, maybe I'd understand how I'm now feeling. Maybe I'd be able to cope better with the nausea, the shaking, the terrible regret.

If I'd listened, maybe I wouldn't be so terrified.

Maybe I'd be able to accept the fact that, in an hour's time, I won't exist.

PART ONE

The Preparation Period

Three months earlier

Amelia

The sessions begin on the first weekend in July. It's uncomfortably hot. The short walk from the van to the Clinic requires me to gather my hair into a ponytail and blot the back of my neck with a tissue.

'I can't believe we're here,' Mum says, tugging at her shirt as we ascend the stone steps leading to the Clinic's entrance. 'Whenever your father and I walked past this place, we'd always speculate about the guests lucky enough to be inside. He'd be so proud of his girls for getting in.'

The Clinic used to be a luxurious hotel, favoured by wealthy tourists due to its proximity to Tower Bridge. The building is imposing, four storeys of elaborate brickwork and Gothic spires. A row of silver flagpoles extends along the roofline. Each one holds a forest-green flag, hanging limp and still in the absence of any breeze.

Mum begins climbing faster, spurred on by her excitement and seemingly unfazed by the heat or the angry shouts of the protestors behind us. Her eyes are fixed on the grand stone carvings of trees flanking the Clinic's large mahogany doors.

Mum and I have already climbed these stone steps, already passed through the Trees of Connection, their mottled grey branches intertwining to form an elegant arch. We visited the Clinic last month for our interviews, but I don't remind her of this. I let her relish the excitement of entering the building for the first time.

A petite woman wearing a plum-coloured tunic greets us at the door. A neat bun, coiled with precision, sits atop her head. She hands us glasses of iced water and peers down the steps at the protestors gathered on the pavement, their placards hoisted high above their heads. 'I hope they didn't bother you too much,' she says, ushering us inside. 'They're relentless in their mission to upset and provoke. I just wish they didn't target innocent people such as yourselves.'

We follow the woman into the large foyer. Our footsteps echo on the marble floor, decorated with swirls of white and grey, the wave-like pattern suggesting the sea. Mum drinks her water, draining the glass, her eyes wide as she takes in the high ceiling. 'Goodness,' she whispers. 'Isn't it remarkable?'

I stand with her as she admires the mural stretching above us, the array of featureless golden figures that intersect and overlap on a black background.

A Combine night sky, Eliza called it.

When we came for our interviews last month, it was Eliza who guided us through the foyer. 'See the scroll in that figure's hand?' She pointed to a golden body sprawled above us. 'It's representative of knowledge. And do you notice the outstretched arms of the figure it's connected to? They symbolise compassion. Each figure embodies a distinctive human quality.' I looked closely and noticed other 'symbols' hidden among the golden figures: a saxophone tucked under an arm, hands resting together in prayer, a pair of ballet shoes. 'It serves as a visual reminder,' Eliza said, 'of the extraordinary power that's bestowed on us when we truly come together.'

Now, the woman in the purple tunic directs our attention to a small figure with closed eyes, their hands gently clasped in meditation. 'Notice,' she says, extending her arm and pointing, 'how the figure beside them, though identical, is alert and awake. Do you see the energy lines connecting them?'

I squint, straining to see the thin, almost imperceptible lines flowing between the figures. Mum tilts her head back further, frowning as she scrutinises the mural. Eventually, she nods. 'Energy lines,' she says, though I doubt she's entirely convinced of their existence.

The woman leads us further into the lobby, towards the large marble statue of Our Combine that stands proudly in the centre of the foyer. Their outstretched hands, smooth and polished, beckon us to join in their mission, to embrace the sacrifice they represent.

An elderly couple dressed in floor-length purple robes pose in front of the statue. A photographer stands a short distance away, a large camera raised to his eye. He must have special permission. Photography, Eliza told me last month when I got my phone out to take a photo, is strictly forbidden.

The elderly couple face one another, holding hands, their arms outstretched. The photographer snaps a few photos, the camera clicking loudly, before directing them to move closer. 'Nose to nose,' he says. 'So close that your vision blurs when you look at one another.' The couple do as instructed. They stand, the tips of their noses touching.

The pose, though regularly used in advertisements, feels uncomfortably intimate to witness in person. Such closeness feels almost sacred, a communion of spirits.

A shared breath passes between the elderly couple.

I look away.

It's possible this photoshoot is purely commercial, and these images are intended for buses and billboards, leaflets for retirement homes at full capacity. But there's a chance it's genuine, and this couple really is about to Commit. If that's the case, witnessing their final moments without the invitation to do so seems intrusive. Indelicate.

We continue past the statue and reach the front desk: a large, curved stone counter behind which three Combine employees, also wearing plum-coloured tunics, sit in front of a low bank of screens. The woman remains standing with us as a man with tight black curls smiles from behind the desk. 'Welcome to the Tower Bridge Clinic. Please could I have the name of your Group Leader?'

'It's Eliza Singh. We're Laurie and Amelia Anderson.' I open my bag and give him our passports, which are already open on the photo page. I read the email explaining what to do once we arrived at the Clinic so many times that I'm sure I could recite it by heart.

1. *Head directly to the Clinic's entrance, where a designated staff member will be ready to welcome you.*

2. *Provide the name of your Group Leader to begin the check-in process.*

3. *Present your identification documents, passports or government-issued IDs to the receptionist. Make sure the photo page is open and clearly visible for verification.*

There were ten instructions in total. I read them obsessively. It was the only tangible evidence I had that this was actually happening. No announcements, no news articles confirmed the commencement date for the trials. They couldn't risk any repercussions.

The man behind the desk continues to smile as he takes and examines our passports. He glances at Mum, who's watching the elderly couple with interest. 'It's best not to stare,' he says gently. 'We want them to enjoy their photoshoot, not feel as though they're being observed.'

I smile apologetically as Mum, taking no notice, continues to watch them. The man doesn't reinforce his suggestion, and I don't try to get Mum to stop staring. We're having a good morning, and I'd like it to remain that way.

He begins inputting our details, his fingers moving quickly over the keyboard. Mounted on the wall behind him is a large golden mandala, a perfect circle split by a curved line shaped like a loose 's'. On either side of the line is the illustration of a brain, one black, the other white. Waves flow between them. I sip my water and consider how many years of experience the tattooists must need to replicate such an intricate pattern on such a small area of skin.

'Though people are physically merging,' Our Combine said during their first televised announcement, 'living as a Combine allows you to celebrate and to utilise the essence of each person's individuality.' The camera panned slowly around them, revealing the tattooed emblem on their neck. 'The mark of a Combine serves as a reminder of the beauty that the Transfer gifts the Host. It is a symbol of balance and interconnection and a reminder of the Combine's astonishing capabilities.'

The man returns our passports along with two name badges. I help Mum pin hers to her shirt before putting mine on. 'You should wear the badges at all times while in the Clinic,' the woman says as she leads us back through the foyer. 'It prevents any misunderstandings about your access within the premises.'

We walk past the statue and the still-posing couple, through a large set of double doors and down a long, well-lit corridor. As we walk, Mum recounts the story she always tells once summer has finally arrived, about an earlier summer when I was seven and it was so cold we still had the heating on in July.

'You can't imagine it,' the woman says politely. 'On days like these, it seems we'll never feel cold again. We're due to hit highs of forty-three again this week. Though it's Italy who seems to be really suffering at the moment. Calabria is on fire again, and they only got Sicily under control a few days ago. The flames were mountainous.'

The radio was playing in the van that brought us here. A devastated woman had called in to talk to the harassed presenter. The woman had been so sure that, come July, the earth would no longer be parched, the plants no longer wilted. The rivers no longer shrunk to streams, their grey beds cracked like cement. She began to cry and was abruptly cut off by music. Mum snorted: 'What did she think, that the weather was just waiting for the calendar to flip before turning from drought to downpour?'

If not for my impatience for the sessions to start, I'd have no real idea how long this heatwave has lasted. June was a blur, the days always too long, eliding into one another, each one indistinguishable from the last.

'Here we are,' the woman says, a hint of relief in her voice. Mum smiles, unfazed by the interruption mid-story. She'd been busy explaining how Dad meticulously applied factor fifty to his ears before leaving the house, even on overcast days. 'Room One,' the woman says, gesturing to the door ahead. 'Right opposite The Oasis, so you won't have to go far for your breaks.'

Room One is small and plain, empty of furniture save for a circle of folding metal chairs set out in the centre. Sitting in the circle are two women and a man, all wearing plum-coloured tunics. 'Your Support Workers,' the woman explains. She gestures at the other six people in the circle, dressed in regular clothes. 'And these are your fellow Participants.'

A lady with curly red hair smiles uncertainly at us. Everyone else avoids eye contact.

Two large windows are covered by thick black blinds. 'For your privacy,' the woman says, following my gaze. 'Reporters are hungry. A shot of the eight of you together would be worthy of the front page. Please, have a seat. Eliza will be joining you shortly.' She bows her head. 'Thank you for your sacrifice.' She leaves the room, closing the door silently behind her.

There are three empty chairs. Two of the vacant seats are together, the other stands alone between four Participants. The Support Workers are seated to divide each pair. 'Is this it?' Mum whispers as we head for the two seats next to each other. 'I was expecting something a lot fancier, weren't you? This feels like a doctor's waiting room.'

She's right. The room has a medical feel about it. It's harshly lit and has the lingering odour of the cleaning products they use to keep the place spotless. It has the charged atmosphere of a doctor's waiting room, too, filled with nervous people expecting bad news. I sit and make the mistake of glancing at the spotlight above me; when I look around the circle again, orbs of light blur my vision, distorting the faces.

Amelia

Eliza enters the room. Her black hair is tightly braided into a ponytail, just as it was during our interview. She makes her way to the vacant chair, completing the pattern of a purple uniform on every third seat. 'Welcome, everybody,' she says. 'It's brilliant to see you all here today. Getting a group together for the first time is always so exciting. As you're aware, these sessions will be taking place weekly. Every Saturday at nine a.m. your group will meet in The Oasis for tea and coffee. This gives you a chance to chat, relax and enjoy one another's company before we begin.'

To my right sits a teenage boy, thin and pale, wearing a beanie the exact same shade of green as his sleeveless top. His eyes are not on Eliza, but me.

'I know it can be daunting meeting the other Participants,' Eliza says, 'but rest assured you'll become much more relaxed as the weeks go on. Over the next three months the eight of you will grow extremely close. You'll get to know one another in a way that is entirely unique to your situation.' She gestures to the group as a whole. 'You start off as strangers and end up as family.'

The boy in the beanie has shifted his attention to Mum. She's writing in her new notebook, the brown leather one I bought her last month. It's smaller than her previous one, pocket-sized, easier for her to carry around. Her pen moves quickly across the page. I resist the urge to reach out and stop her. I've explained so many times that she should limit her notes and record only the most important information. She never listens.

'What I'd like to do is go around the circle and introduce ourselves.' Eliza rests her hand on her chest. 'I know you've already met me, but for the purpose of this exercise, let's assume you haven't. I'm Eliza Singh. I'm a psychiatrist, and I've been working for Combine for five years. My job is to lead your group sessions, to provide support and offer guidance.' She pauses, taking the time to look at each of us. When our eyes meet, I offer a small smile. 'The eight of you are going above and beyond the usual sacrifice asked of our Participants. By volunteering to partake in an Experimental Merge, you are making the ultimate leap of faith, and I applaud you for your courage and compassion. I know for a fact that my admiration is echoed by each member of our team.'

The Support Workers nod in agreement.

Eliza turns to the couple sitting to her left: the red-haired woman who smiled at us earlier and a man of a similar age with short dark hair and a small diamond stud in his nose. 'Why don't we start with you two? Please introduce yourselves to the group. Tell us your names, ages, a little about yourselves and why you're here.'

The couple look at one another. The woman's hands are tucked between her thighs, and her partner, with his fingers interlocked, looks equally apprehensive. He raises his hand. 'I'm Ben,' he says. 'I'm thirty-two, and a circular economy strategist. This lovely young lady sitting next to me is my fiancée, Annie.'

Annie laughs, embarrassed. She has a round face, her cheeks flushed with generously applied blusher. 'Sorry,' she says, covering her mouth. 'I'm terrible at things like this. I never know what to say.'

Eliza smiles, and I find myself smiling too. I lift my chin in an attempt to mimic her posture. There's something regal about Eliza, something superior in the way she holds herself.

'How old are you, Annie?' Eliza asks. 'And what do you do for a living?'

'I'm twenty-eight and I'm a physio. I do stroke rehab.'

'And why are the two of you here today?'

Ben and Annie share another look. He reaches for her hand. 'Annie's pregnant,' he says.

I tense, preparing for the uncomfortable silence that often follows a pregnancy announcement, but Eliza begins clapping, as do the Support Workers. The rest of us quickly join in. Beside me, Mum puts down her pen to clap properly.

Ben smiles appreciatively, still holding Annie's hand.

Annie keeps her gaze on her lap. She doesn't smile. She doesn't look up until the attention shifts to the Support Worker sitting next to her. When Annie eventually looks at him, I notice her eyes are startlingly blue. And that they're wet.

'Hi.' The Support Worker smiles, his long legs stretched out in front of him, crossed at the ankle. 'I'm Nathan. I'm fifty, a dad of two beautiful girls, Isla and Georgie, and I've been doing this for three years now. Before working for Combine, I was a psychotherapist. I worked predominantly with patients who suffered from schizophrenia. I did that for over two decades.'

'Schizophrenia,' Mum mutters, writing quickly.

'Because of my background, I understand how traumatic it can be not knowing whether you can trust your thoughts. I'm here to prepare you, to teach you how to cope, should that situation ever arise.'

Again, Eliza claps and the rest of us join in.

Next in the circle is the boy in the beanie. He sits beside a younger boy with strawberry-blond hair. There's an uncomfortable silence. The boy in the beanie stares ahead at nothing while the younger one looks at him expectantly. I pick at a loose thread on my dress until, eventually, the younger one speaks. 'Hi,' he says, 'I'm Lucas and…' He looks again at the boy in the beanie. 'This is my brother, Noah. I'm fifteen and Noah's seventeen. We're both still in school. At least we were, but, well…' Lucas pauses. Noah remains silent. 'Noah's… Noah's got leukaemia. He's been in remission twice, but it's come back again and it's worse this time. That's why we're here. To make Noah better.'

We don't wait for Eliza this time. We clap, more enthusiastically than we have done so far. Lucas nods in recognition of our applause and Nathan puts a hand on Noah's shoulder. Mum and I look at each other.

The Support Worker sitting between Lucas and me waits for the applause to fade. 'Hi, everyone,' she says and smiles. 'I'm Callie. I'm forty-four and a licensed therapist. Prior to becoming a Support Worker I helped my brother, Rosa-Liam, go through the Merge. They were enrolled in a much larger group. It was back in the early days when the Merge was first being rolled out. Rosa-Liam's group didn't have access to the level of support that we enjoy now. I believe there were also three Support Workers in their cohort. Three Support Workers for sixty-odd Participants.' She shakes her head. 'Through helping Rosa-Liam, I discovered how important it is that people who are in your position are fully supported. I'm honoured to be part of this group. I so admire each of you for being here.'

Everybody claps. Then all eyes focus on us.

I reach over and gently close Mum's notebook.

'Hi,' I say, smiling my way around the circle. 'I'm Amelia and this is my mum, Laurie. I'm twenty-three and Mum's sixty-five.' I take Mum's hand, aware of how she might feel with all these strangers' eyes on her. I wait, in case she wants to speak, but she's not looking at me. She's staring intently at the others. 'I'm a wedding videographer, primarily,' I say, 'though I do a lot of Commitment Ceremonies now. Mum is – was – a teacher. She's dedicated her life to teaching children with special educational needs.' I smile and give Mum's hand a squeeze. She's frowning at the faces, hating the attention. 'She's incredible... Her work has helped hundreds of children. But sadly, Mum now has Alzheimer's. It's just the two of us. Dad died during the climate protests almost ten years ago. So that's... that's why we're here, really.'

Mum lets go of my hand. She claps along with everyone else.

I struggle to concentrate as the next Support Worker introduces herself. She's Angela, a physio, and she'll be working predominantly with the Hosts. Beyond that, I don't hear much. I watch Mum as she listens. She hates people knowing about her illness. She does everything she can to hide it, and here I am, announcing her secret to a roomful of strangers as though it's common knowledge. It's necessary, but that doesn't make it any easier.

I gather myself in time to hear the final Participants, Jay and Lara, introduce themselves. They're father and daughter. 'I'm from India originally,' Jay says. 'I moved to England because I met Kath, Lara's mother, at a business convention here in London. We're both management consultants. Lara's a student.' He looks at his daughter, but she offers nothing. 'She's an addict,' he says softly.

Lara looks at the floor, her hair falling over her shoulders, as Jay tells us about her struggles with drugs. She's dressed in a thick, oversized black hoodie. Her slouched posture makes her look tiny. Her father, bald and wearing a shirt and tie, sits upright, his legs spread.

'I'm one hundred and six days clean,' Lara says once her dad has finished telling their story. 'But he doesn't trust me to stay that way.'

Jay swallows, remains composed. 'Lara's addiction has robbed her of any stability,' he says. 'She's only seventeen and she has so much potential. I just want to help my beautiful daughter get back on track.'

There's more clapping. Mum returns to her notetaking.

Laurie

It is unfathomably difficult to know what's right, to know whether I should even be entertaining Amelia's curiosity regarding us 'merging'. Mary insists the decision is simple. She is categorically against my being here, convinced that I am providing Amelia with false hope and doing her no favours. She argues that I should be honest about my reservations, that Amelia will understand why I don't want to merge, and that she'll cope.

But Amelia has a tendency not to cope. She's always been the same. Ever since she was a little girl, she's confronted unwelcome news with denial. When she accidentally tore the wing of her beloved stuffed penguin, Waddles, I braced myself for the flood of tears. But she didn't cry. She placed Waddles among her pillows and smiled, declaring he was 'resting after a flight'. When the police officers turned up at the house and delivered the horrific news about Mitchell's death, Amelia stared at them, quiet and expressionless. She didn't break down as I did. She went upstairs and tidied her room. 'Dad hates it when it's messy,' she said when I asked what she was doing. 'He'll be cross if I don't sort it out.'

It's how she is: defiant, as if her resistance alone can render something untrue. If she'd accepted my diagnosis, if she'd come to terms with the progressive nature of my disease, she'd never have applied for this experiment. Applying was, in itself, an act of rebellion. Everyone told her there was no cure for Alzheimer's. So she found one.

As everyone files out of the room for lunch, I slip my notebook into my bag and attempt to stand, but Amelia puts her hand on my arm, stopping me. 'Wait, Mum. How was that for you?'

'Good,' I tell her. 'Interesting. Can we eat now?'

'You're feeling okay?'

'Yes, Amelia. I'm fine, but I'm hungry.'

Her eyes, wide and searching, hold mine. She does this, performs silent interrogations, hunts for something I'm not saying, reaches for the words I've chosen not to speak. I hold her stare, steady and unwavering, until – finally – her expression softens. A smile. 'Okay,' she says. 'Good. Let's get some lunch.'

It's a strange thing to come to terms with, being parented by your daughter. I did the same for my mother, always watching over her, unable to relax until she was right there in front of me and I knew she was safe. I don't believe my mother was aware of the responsibility I felt as a child and was thus unburdened by it, but for me the opposite is true. Every time I catch Amelia worrying about me, I am reminded of the weight of nurturing that falls on the shoulders of young caregivers. A heritable pattern I so wish had ended with me.

I wait for Amelia to gather herself. She takes her time, observing the room as though the white walls and metal chairs are of interest to her. She's stalling, readying herself to question me again, to check I really *am* okay. I quickly leave the room and wait for her in the corridor.

There's a sign mounted on the wall, *The Oasis,* engraved on a polished brass plaque. I trace the curled lettering with a finger. 'An oasis,' my mother would say, the tips of her forefingers pressed to the tips of her thumbs. 'A respite from chaos.'

I'd smile, delighted by what was to come. It wasn't often that my stepfather was out. We'd savour the rare moment of freedom, quickly falling into hysterics, the two of us high on his absence. 'He's a good man really,' my mother would say during her inevitable comedown, caused by me questioning why she remained married to him when she was so much happier in his absence. She'd wince, and I'd not know if it was my words that had stung her or the cut on her lip, reopened during her laughter. 'I wouldn't have picked him otherwise.'

I push the memory away. Let it linger, and I'll become stuck there. Distant memories pull me in, preferable, even with the pain they bring, to the present; the moments from years gone so much more solid than those happening now; so much easier to make sense of. As though my childhood happened just yesterday, and yesterday a lifetime ago.

Amelia appears from the other room. She smiles. 'All okay?'

I nod, and she opens the door to The Oasis, revealing a large room with high corniced ceilings and a green marbled floor, the pattern resembling waterweed. A young girl with dark hair sits alone at a long oak refectory table, her back to the glass wall overlooking the Thames. She slumps forward, shoulders rounded, idly scoring the wood with her nail. Behind her, others from our group look through the glass at the river. The two boys stand together, whispering. The bald man in the suit and tie chats with the young couple, their arms looped round each other's waists. The woman wears a pale-yellow dress dotted with small white circles. The hem is uneven, as though it has been stitched by her own hand.

Mary was always making clothes, using me as her mannequin. 'Honestly,' I'd say, shifting restlessly under her incessant measuring. 'I can buy a top. You don't need to make one.'

Mary would continue rolling up my cuffs, running the tape measure round my waist, holding swatches of fabrics against my skin, a needle invariably gripped between her teeth. 'I know I don't need to make it,' she'd say. 'I want to. I'm going to sew my soul into the fabric.'

'Your soul?' I'd pause, allow only the faintest smile to touch my lips. 'Well then, I guess it's never coming off.'

She'd nod, the needle bobbing with her words. 'Exactly as planned. Consider it my way of wrapping you in a hug every day.'

Amelia has joined the others by the window. There's a storm coming in, the dark clouds piling up on top of each other. She presses her palms to the glass, eyes fixed on the bridge. I move to stand beside her, and together we look at the flattened view of London, squashed like a pancake.

'Beautiful, isn't it?'

She nods, not looking away. Only when she begins muttering, willing the impending downpour, do I realise it's not the bridge that excites her – it's the weather. I step back, suddenly aware of the relentless weeks of sun I'd almost forgotten.

Amelia turns from the window. 'What is it? What's wrong?'

I force a smile. 'Why don't we play the game you loved as a child?' I suggest. 'Where we find letters of the alphabet in our surroundings.' I point out the 'H' shape of Tower Bridge, blocked with traffic. 'Let's see how many other letters we can find. The Shard could be a capital "I".'

But Amelia doesn't want to play. 'We should eat,' she says, turning away from the view. 'We haven't got long before the sessions start again.'

Amelia was little when Mitchell introduced the alphabet game. The memory remains vivid despite the blur of time: we were walking in the rain, exploring Bourne Woods with our hoods up and wellington boots on. I can still picture the exact ridge we were standing on when Mitchell pointed out the letter 'M' in the shape of a blackbird's wings. I'd thought him silly to expect Amelia to find any letters, until she picked up a fallen leaf and pointed at the 'L' traced in its veins.

There's a crash of thunder. A deluge of rain.

A cheer and laughter. Amelia's no less delighted now than she was when she found the leaf. I sit opposite her at the table, beside the dark-haired girl, who slumps in her chair, staring moodily at her empty glass, completely uninterested in the rain pouring down behind her, creating a curtain of silver.

'Can I top you up?' I offer.

The girl doesn't look up, doesn't acknowledge me as I refill her glass. When a plate of pasta is placed in front of her by a man in a purple tunic, she doesn't offer so much as a grunt. 'Thank you,' I say when I'm handed a ciabatta sandwich with a green salad. I smile, but Amelia senses my disappointment.

'You said you wanted the mozzarella and pesto sandwich, Mum. I told you that you'd change your mind, but you insisted you wouldn't.'

'Quite right,' I say, taking a bite. 'This is just what I fancy.'

I make a mental note to order the pasta next week.

As I eat, I tune in to the snippets of conversation happening along the table. 'Did you ever think we'd be cheering about rain?' the young, short-haired man is saying. 'I know it's only been a few weeks, but I'd almost forgotten what it looked like. Has it always been this epic?' Further down the table, the freckly-faced boy chatters on about his girlfriend. 'We met in big band in Year Eight. I play trombone. Ellie plays the flute. We didn't start properly dating until last year.' Their conversations do nothing to aid my memory. Try as I might, I can't recall any of their names.

Another crash of thunder. Another cheer. More laughter. The girl beside me pulls up her hood, shadowing her face as she pushes pasta around her plate with her fork.

'Why do some people have pasta, Amelia? I'd have liked pasta.'

'You said you wanted a sandwich, Mum.'

'Did I?'

'Yes.'

The woman in the yellow dress smiles kindly at me from across the table. I return her smile and reach into my bag for my notebook. I've dedicated a page to each Participant and sketched them alongside their name. I flip through the pages until I land on the one I'm looking for – the sketch of the curly-haired girl. There she is. Annie. I run my finger along the notes.

'What are you smiling about?' Amelia asks, eyeing my notebook.

'She's pregnant,' I whisper.

Amelia nods. 'That's why they're here.'

'How lovely.' I daren't reveal my excitement at the prospect of having a pregnant friend. Amelia has always found my interest in pregnancy irritating. When she was younger, she used to get embarrassed whenever I made a fuss over a baby bump. I remember one particular encounter with her pregnant teacher, a funny woman with a bad temper and a strong distaste for Amelia's self-righteousness. It was parents' evening, and I was introducing myself to the bump. Amelia, mortified, told me off. 'It can't hear you,' she snapped. 'Stop talking to it.'

Now that pregnancy is no longer celebrated, Amelia's all the more embarrassed by my interest. I sometimes forget that people no longer welcome new life with any sense of joy, and it gets me into trouble. Women think I'm shaming them, congratulating them ironically. 'Just walk past them, Mum,'

Amelia says whenever she catches me looking at a pregnant stomach. 'Behave like a normal person.'

We go through my notebook together. Amelia quietly admires the sketches while I reacquaint myself with everyone's stories: pregnancy, cancer, addiction. When I finally close the book and glance down the table, I'm filled with such sadness.

'Not hungry?' I ask the girl next to me.

I check her name badge: *Lara, Participant.*

'Not hungry, Lara?'

She shrugs.

I take another bite of my sandwich. It's important to eat. If nothing else, it means I avoid Amelia's wrath.

'How old are you?' I ask after a while.

'Seventeen,' she says. 'Nine months too young to have a choice about being here.'

'You don't want to be here?'

'Fuck, no. Do you?'

I turn to watch the still-torrential rain, listening as Amelia chats to the man sitting beside her. They're predicting what we'll be doing after lunch. More of the same, he thinks. Finding out how it all works, Amelia hopes. I wait until they're deep in conversation, then lean towards Lara.

'Truth be told,' I whisper, 'I don't want to be here either.'

Lara looks at me. 'Really?'

I nod.

'Why are you here, then?'

'Amelia thinks it's for the best. She's struggling, you see, to come to terms with my diagnosis.'

'Jesus.' Lara puts her fork down. 'I thought my dad was the only person psychotic enough to force somebody into this.'

'She isn't forcing me. She's just worried.' I glance at Amelia to ensure she's not listening. 'I have three months to decide if it's right for me.'

'You're lucky you get a choice,' Lara says.

I frown. 'Don't you have a choice?'

'No.'

'Why not?'

'Under eighteen. I have no say. It's totally fucked up.'

I stare at her. I must have known about the under-eighteen rule. Someone must have told me – Amelia, probably. I close my eyes, willing the memory to resurface. It's exhausting, trying to remember, trying to make sense of it all.

'Laurie? Are you okay?'

I open my eyes to find the young girl has lowered her hood. Her features have softened with her concern. 'I'm just trying to remember,' I say. 'It sometimes helps when I close my eyes. It shuts everything else out.'

'That must be scary,' she says. 'Forgetting things.'

'It must be scary having no say in things, too. You know, Lara, my mother struggled with addiction. I'm so terribly sorry that you're suffering.'

Something flashes across her face. Embarrassment, I think. Anger, too.

I finish my sandwich and open my bag. I add a note in my notebook.

Under 18s have no choice.

Laurie

It's a relief to be home.

Amelia sits in the armchair opposite me, already in her pyjamas despite it still being daylight. The bottoms stop halfway down her calves, badly faded, the yellow bird faces barely visible. She was obsessed with that little bird. Tweetie Pie, I think it's called. There was a cat too. Her phone is pointed at me. I smile. She's forever taking photos. I dread to think how many thousands she has on her phone. I'd like to get them printed, to sit down and look at them together properly. She's such a gifted photographer. Mitchell always said so.

She laughs at my frozen smile. 'It's a video, Mum,' she says. 'I wanted to document our first day. How are you feeling after the first session? The group seem nice, don't they?'

I let my smile soften. 'Yes,' I say, although I have no real idea. I remember some faces from the session – the pregnant girl with the curly red hair, the poorly boy in the hat – but I can't recall if they were nice.

It doesn't get any easier, the realisation that I've forgotten something. As soon as I notice, it's impossible to leave the forgotten thing alone. The missing details nag at my mind. It's like reading a book and skipping a page, a paragraph, a chapter. I continue with the story, but a part of me is distracted, wondering what I've missed, wondering whether things would be different if I knew what had happened on those unread pages.

I reach for my notebook, but Amelia stops me. 'Don't, Mum,' she says. 'It's been a really long day. Let yourself relax.'

My fingers brush the notebook before I pick up my mug from the coffee table. Amelia's right. I mustn't worry. I take a sip of tea. It's horribly weak. She probably let the bag sit in the water for just a few seconds before transferring it to the bin.

Like many people, Amelia believes caffeine worsens Alzheimer's symptoms. I don't buy into it. Mitchell and I gave up eating food that came in a tin for years before it was conclusively proved that canned food had no link to cancer. When I realised it was all nonsense, I celebrated by eating so many tins of peaches that I had to lie still on the sofa for fear of being sick.

I yawn, and Amelia smiles, putting her phone down. 'I imagine the sessions will become less tiring as the weeks go on.' She picks up her mug – Mitchell's mug. Red with black spots, like a ladybird. For a long time, I kept the mug hidden away. I can't think when I brought it out again. Perhaps it was Amelia who found it. Though she rarely talks about her father, she finds other ways to keep him close: listening to his vinyl collection and watching *Grand Designs*, even though she doesn't care much for jazz or architecture. Drinking from his mug.

Mitchell loved ladybirds. He always made a point of counting the dots on their wing cases, favouring the ones with unequal markings. 'It makes them singularly uncommon,' he'd say as the asymmetrical ladybird crawled over his hand. 'That's the beauty, Lor. How dull would the world be if we were all the same?'

'Did you read the brochure?' Amelia asks.

I shake my head, though I'm not entirely sure. I may well have read a brochure, may well have finished a novel just yesterday, but I can't recall. 'What was it about?'

Amelia sets Mitchell's mug down and leaves the room, her pale legs visible in the gaps between her socks and her too-small pyjama bottoms. I take a sip of tea. It's horribly weak. My eyes linger on the ladybird mug, tempted to taste her drink and see if it's as flavourless as mine. Amelia's always had a distaste for overpowering flavours. 'Too much pepper,' she'd say, wrinkling her nose and pushing away the plate of scrambled eggs.

I wonder how that would work if we went through with the Merge. Whose taste would we inherit? Whose would dominate? I don't like the thought of a life devoid of flavour.

Amelia returns, brochure in hand. She passes it to me. 'See what you think. The statistics might put your mind at ease.'

'I'm not worried,' I say.

'I heard you telling Lara you weren't happy about being there.'

'I—'

'I get it, Mum. It's... weird for me too. Just have a read. It made me feel better.' She settles back into the armchair, tucking her legs under her as she picks up her phone again. 'Honestly, Mum. It might help.'

I open the booklet.

<u>The Merge: Unlock the Potential</u>
<u>of a Unified Consciousness</u>

Unprecedented 99% Reduction in Existential Anxiety: Combines report a groundbreaking 99% decrease in existential anxiety, demonstrating the transformative impact of shared consciousness on existential concerns.
80% Rise in Job Performance Ratings: Combine professionals receive an impressive 80%

boost in job performance ratings, suggesting that shared skills and collective problem-solving lead to heightened workplace efficiency.

We sit quietly for a while, me pretending to read, Amelia smiling at me between sips of tea. It's the same sympathetic smile I used to give my mother, and it hurts. I close the brochure.

'Who are you doing this "merging" for?' I ask.

She frowns. 'For us.'

'For me, you mean?'

'No, Mum. Us.'

She offers another patronising smile. I swallow, sinking beneath the waves of her sympathy.

'Is Albie coming over?'

'No,' she says. 'Not today.'

I watch her as she drinks, her face freshly cleaned, her hair frizzy from brushing. There's a crease between her eyebrows. I'm sure it's new, though how can I be sure? How can I possibly trust myself to know what's changed? There's something different, but I can't pinpoint what exactly.

'What?' she says, the crease deepening.

'You can't waste your life worrying about me, Amelia. You should be out in the world, living your life. Making a life for yourself with Albie. Not holed up at home with me.'

She scoops her hair into a bun and stretches her neck. 'Let's have a patience practice,' she says. 'It'll be good for the both of us.'

'Remember to keep your body relaxed.' Amelia gently repositions my hands to rest on my thighs, palms facing upwards.

'I do remember.' I wiggle my shoulders to release the tension.

'Are you comfy, Mum?'

I nod, though I am far from comfortable. We're sitting, as always, on the rug in the lounge. I'm perched on a cushion, but it doesn't do much by way of support. It's not my bottom that aches during these 'patience practices', as Amelia calls them, but my legs. I'd hoped, when we first started, that sitting cross-legged would become easier over time. It hasn't.

Amelia discovered the exercises online. 'A Combine was signed off less than four months after their Merge,' she'd said, handing me the printed instructions. 'They swore that it was because of these exercises. I think we should try it, Mum.'

I only agreed on account of how strong-willed Amelia is when it comes to my health. Arguing with her would only have delayed the inevitable.

'Good,' she says, settling into position opposite me. She doesn't need a cushion.

She inhales deeply. I do the same.

We release our breath together.

Amelia begins to roll her head gently in a clockwise direction. I mirror her. We start with small, barely noticeable rotations. As we slowly increase our movements, our heads tilt towards the ceiling, the wall, and eventually the floor. Then Amelia reverses direction, moving her head anticlockwise. Gradually the rotations slow until we return to where we started, making delicate movements with our necks until, eventually, we stop altogether.

Amelia exhales and closes her eyes.

This, I don't copy.

The truth is, as much as Amelia wants to help, sitting in silence with an empty mind doesn't benefit me. My time is much better spent working my brain. Thanks to Amelia's focus, her unwillingness to open her eyes and peek even for a moment, these 'patience practices' allow me to do just that.

I scan the room.

As with the rest of the apartment, the lounge is uninspiring. The walls are a faded white, dirtied by the previous owners, and showing the ghosts of long-since-removed pictures. I must have been living here for years now and I've not so much as changed the colour of the curtains. They remain a dull beige, perfect for a home devoid of vibrancy. I say home, but I don't mean it. Though I live here, this is not, and will never be, my home.

Home was with Mitchell. A three-bed cottage with a garden and much laughter. Far from dull. The lounge walls were canary yellow.

I look at the worn sofa that came with the apartment, its faux leather peeling, its once-cushioned seats now sunken. Three navy-blue cushions rest there, slightly askew. Were Mitchell here, he would rearrange them immediately, insisting on their perfect alignment.

There's the ladybird mug on the coffee table. Dust-covered candles in the fireplace. The photograph of Mitchell on the mantelpiece beside the wilting sunflowers from Amelia's birthday. The main light is off. The lamp next to the armchair is lit. Amelia's lilac dressing gown is draped over the back of the armchair. The brown armchair.

I close my eyes.

Amelia is silent as, I suppose, is her mind.

My mind works hard, cataloguing what I've just seen.

When the details are safely stored, I stop and count to a hundred.

Then I begin again.

There was the sofa with the cushions. There were three cushions, and they were blue. Navy blue. There was the coffee table, the ladybird mug. The fireplace. The candles. The sunflowers, dying. Mitchell's photograph. The armchair. The... Wasn't there something on the armchair? I scrunch up my face, willing my brain to retrieve what I can't quite reach. There was definitely something on the armchair. Something blue. A cushion? No, that was on the sofa. A jumper? Yes. But not blue. Green. A green jumper. That was it.

I open my eyes.

My stomach drops at the sight of Amelia's lilac dressing gown.

Amelia

There's mould on Albie's bathroom ceiling, a growing mural of damp that I always forget about until I'm here in the shower, my head tilted back, rinsing shampoo from my hair.

The water burns my scalp, but I don't adjust the temperature. I scrub myself with an exfoliating mitt, rubbing vigorously at my skin until it stings, until my arms and legs ache beneath the scorching water, sore enough to warrant tears.

I shouldn't have come here. I knew what would happen. There was no way I'd come to Albie's and not end up fucking him. I'd been here for minutes, not long enough for Albie to finish pouring us each a glass of wine, when I was kissing him, and he was raising his eyebrows, his lips against mine as I took the bottle from him so that he could hold me properly. We fucked right there against the counter, too hungry for each other to fully undress or make it to the bedroom. Then it was over. I came to my senses while he was still inside me, my dress still bunched in his hands, resting on my hips. I pulled away, tugged my dress down and made for the bathroom, desperate to get clean.

I turn off the water and step out of the shower.

I don't bother to dry myself properly, and my dress clings uncomfortably to my damp skin. I wipe the condensation from the bathroom mirror and use my towel to remove the dark streaks of mascara. My hair drips onto my dress as I leave the bathroom, trailing water as I walk slowly down the narrow corridor towards the lounge. I run my fingers along the walls, resisting the urge to peel at the flaking paint.

The lounge is empty. The low armchair with its geometric motifs sits vacant beside the high-backed wooden chair and the worn recliner. It took Albie months to acquire the seating. All the furnished non-Combine housing was taken, so he had to source everything himself. He spent countless hours hanging around charity shops, waiting for donations. So often when he finally got his hands on a piece of furniture, someone more in need would come along, and he'd end up giving it to them.

I remember the moment Albie realised charity shops were his only option. He was sitting on the floor of his empty lounge, back against the wall, scrolling through a home essentials website. 'The tax is equal to the cost of the chair.' His voice was flat, disbelieving. 'Unless you're a Combine, in which case there is no tax. None.' He looked up at me. 'No wonder the fuckers are doing it.'

There's no sign of Albie in the dining room either. A pile of books sits on the table: *Reclaiming the Wild*, *Environmental Harmony*, *Voices from the Frontlines*. Scattered among the books are sheets of paper covered in scribbled notes and highlighted passages. I resist reading what Albie's written. It would only make everything harder.

The day Albie found the dining table, he called me from the charity shop. 'It's perfect,' he said. 'And it's all mine.' I went to help him carry it home and frowned at the badly chipped top. Albie smiled, his enthusiasm undimmed by my reaction. We carried the damaged table the twenty-minute walk back, and Albie spoke of his plan to upcycle it. We spent evenings and weekends sitting together, cutting ceramic tiles and carefully arranging them into a spiral pattern. In the end, it turned out perfect. Just like Albie said it would.

'I'm in the bedroom,' Albie calls out. 'The fan's in here,' he adds quickly, the way he might have done early on in our relationship, providing an innocent reason to get me into the bedroom.

The lights are off. I turn them on. They flicker, the way they always do before deciding if they'll play ball. Albie's lying on top of the duvet, wearing only his boxers. His mattress sits on a base of repurposed pallets. I join him on the bed. He stretches for the wine glass on his bedside table, his stomach muscles taut as he moves.

'Here.' He hands me the glass. We both prefer red but agreed a couple of summers ago that our taste was going to have to come second to the fact you can add ice to white wine. I thank him and take a sip. Albie watches. He doesn't look away or soften his gaze when I lower the glass and meet his eyes. 'How come you agreed to come over?' he says.

'I don't know,' I say quietly.

I needed to escape the apartment. Mum was following me around with her notebook, asking questions I didn't want to answer. Some of them I couldn't answer. 'What happens to the families who can't afford the taxes?' she asked, her finger resting on a bullet point toward the bottom of the list we'd worked our way through. We'd written the list together after she'd talked to Ben and Annie about their decision to start a family.

Families are required to pay a significant tax (up to £15,000 P/A) for each child they have. Her writing was loopy and slanted, each letter falling into the next like toppled dominos. She kept squinting at the page, certain she'd misread her notes.

'That depends if anyone in the family is willing to merge.' It was a struggle to keep my voice calm. She'd started her questioning over an hour earlier and hadn't written down any of my answers. We'd have to go through it all again when she inevitably forgot everything I'd told her.

'If they all refuse to merge, then what happens?'

'It depends on the circumstances, Mum.'

She waited, her finger still resting on the bullet point.

I sighed. 'If the sum owed is relatively small, you won't be entitled to healthcare,' I said eventually. 'Or education or employment, until the taxes are paid. If it's a larger amount, or if there's very little likelihood of paying it back, you'll probably be forced into merging with someone else who hasn't paid their taxes.'

I turned away, unable to watch her absorb, for what she would believe to be the first time, the realities of the class divide that have taken over the UK. I didn't have the energy to explain how the wealthy are able to maintain their individuality, keep their homes and their families, while the poor are being stripped of everything, forced into a shared existence.

When I finally looked back at her, she was biting her lower lip, tugging at her necklace. 'I don't want to do this,' she said quietly. 'I know I said I'd give it three months, but I don't see myself changing my mind, Amelia. Not when the consequences of all this "merging" are so dire for so many.'

'Give it time, Mum. We don't know all the facts yet. We don't have the full picture.'

She opened her mouth to reply, but I cut her off with a quick kiss on the cheek. 'I love you, Mum,' I said, heading for the door. 'I'm off to see Albie.'

Albie's staring out of the window, his low mattress offering a clear view of the sky.

'Thank you,' I say quietly. 'For everything.'

He nods, turning the stem of his wine glass between his finger and thumb, his eyes fixed on something beyond the glass. 'Have you reconsidered?'

'No,' I say, my voice barely more than a whisper. 'Nothing's changed. I just... I missed you. I'm sorry.'

We sit in silence, the room thick with heat, the only relief coming in the brief, teasing moments when the fan's cool air brushes past us.

My wet hair has nearly dried by the time Albie finally looks at me.

'Why are you doing it?'

'For Mum.' The lie rolls off my tongue, rehearsed so many times it almost sounds convincing.

He sets his glass down, his breath escaping in a low whistle. I know what he wants to ask, the question he's asked so many times since I first told him: *What about me?*

'I'm sorry,' I whisper, my throat tightening. 'I'm so sorry, Albie. I shouldn't have come.'

I waited until the day of my interview with Eliza to break the news to Albie about the Merge. I'd tried to tell him earlier, but the words wouldn't come. Then, with only a month until the sessions began, I had no choice but to come out with it.

'Fuck off.' Albie half-smiled, his face a strange blend of incredulity and concern. We were sitting at his table, the plates in front of us still covered in crumbs from the toast we'd been eating when I blurted out, mouth still full, what I was planning to do.

I used the licked tip of my finger to gather some of the crumbs.

'You're not serious,' he said, eyes narrowing. 'You're joking, right?'

I shook my head. 'I'm not joking, Albie.'

Albie stared, waiting for a smile, for some sign that I was

messing with him. 'You're going to combine with your mum? You're going to voluntarily give yourself up for the Merge?'

I nodded.

He rested his hand on mine, the smile fading. 'Your mum's sick, Amelia. I get that you don't want her to be. I get that it's the most fucking unfair thing in the world to watch her like this, but you can't... Merging with her won't... She has Alzheimer's, Amelia.'

'And this trial is for Alzheimer's patients,' I said. 'It's a potential cure, Albie. It would mean Mum could get herself back, that I could bring my mum back.'

He squeezed my hand. 'This isn't just about you and your mum, Amelia. It's about every family torn apart, every person forced into this system who never had a choice. It's people losing themselves, losing each other.' He looked away, and then back at me, his face open, vulnerable. 'You'd be walking into the very thing we've fought against. What was all that work for? All your research... You'd be giving up everything. Everything we've worked towards – everything we are.' He paused, swallowing hard. 'What about us?'

'Nothing would have to change between us,' I said, fighting to keep my voice steady. 'Lots of people remain in relationships once merged. We could—'

'Bullshit.' He pulled his hand away. 'Relationships don't survive the Merge. If you do this, it means we can't be together. You *know* that.'

I stared down at the tabletop, at the spiral of ceramic tiles, and noticed a discoloured tile disrupting the pattern.

'You know the odds of us still loving each other after you merge are smaller than winning the lottery, right? Or, say we did stay together, if by some miracle the new version of you loved me, and I loved it, we could never Commit. You'd already be Committed to someone else.'

'I thought you never wanted to merge.'

'I don't. Fuck, no. But if things keep going the way they are… maybe someday it won't be a choice anymore. And if that day comes, I'd want to merge with you, Amelia. No one else. I can't do that if you've already merged with your mum.'

I looked up at him. His face. Pale and twisted. I reached for his hand, and this time he let me take it. 'Albs, listen. There's a very real chance that, this time next year, Mum won't know who I am. I can stop that from happening. I can make sure I never lose her. I've already lost Dad. I can't be an orphan at twenty-three.'

'She'll still be there, Amelia. She's not dying, she's just…'

I waited, watching him.

'She's changing,' he finished.

'Forgetting,' I corrected him. 'Forgetting who she is, where she is, how to behave. Forgetting everything. I have a chance to stop her forgetting, Albs. I have a chance to save my mum, to not have to say goodbye.'

He stared at me, silence stretching between us.

'What about you?' he said finally. 'The risks of the trials – everyone knows them. They're not some vague threat. You could lose your mind, Amelia, take on her Alzheimer's.'

I looked down at our hands, his still resting in mine.

'I know,' I said.

'And you're okay with that? You'll risk losing your mind, forgetting everything, at the age of twenty-three? You're willing to wake up one day and not know who you are, who I am, who anyone is?'

'If it means saving Mum,' I said, my voice barely a whisper, 'then yes.'

His face tightened. 'But what about us? Amelia, if you do this you're saying goodbye to us, too.'

I shook my head, forcing the words through the ache in my

throat. 'I already said, nothing would have to change.'

He pulled his hand back sharply, smacking the table so hard that the plates rattled. 'Everything would have to change. *You're* the person I love, Amelia. Not some fucking warped version that's half you and half your mum.' His face contorted. 'We could never have sex again. There's no way I'm fucking you with your mum in there. How will you ever fuck anyone? Think about it, Amelia. If you do this, you're not just saying goodbye to me. You're saying goodbye to sex completely.' He leaned forward, his voice lower, pleading. 'But if *we* merged... if we Committed properly... We could feel what each other are feeling. We could have sex together, like, actually together.'

'With someone else?'

Albie shrugged. 'I guess. Or just us. We'd have options. If you merge with your mum, Amelia, you have no options. None.'

'I know,' I said.

'So, think about it.' Albie's voice softened. 'Don't just do this to be a martyr. Really think about it. Think about what you'd be giving up.' He leaned close, his eyes wide. 'Think about us.'

Amelia

The protestors are silent this morning, their placards held high above their heads, their mouths unmoving. Despite my instruction to keep her eyes lowered, Mum reads their signs.

I knew there wouldn't be any shouting today; I saw on the news that the protestors have changed tack. 'Anti-Mergers have declared a month-long silence,' the reporter announced, 'in solidarity for those whose voices, they say, are being taken from them. In a statement released at eleven last night, an Anti-Merge spokesman explained their mission to stand silent with the Transfers, whose rights, they claim, are obliterated the moment they merge. Their vow of silence will begin at midnight and extend until the end of July.'

There's a slight breeze. The wind tugs at my hair as I climb the steps to the Clinic. The flags flutter lazily. Mum trails behind, yawning loudly. Neither of us slept well last night. The heat felt thicker than usual, impossible to ignore. I lay awake into the early hours, listening to Mum's restless pacing, the floorboards creaking beneath her feet.

'What time did you finally get to sleep?' I ask, slipping my arm through hers as we cross the foyer towards the front desk. 'It must have been late. I heard you in the kitchen at two.'

Mum waves a dismissive hand. 'You know how I am these days. It's all the blasted medication, muddling my mind. I'm sleepy all day, but come night-time I suddenly feel wide awake.'

We sign in and make our way to The Oasis. As we walk through the foyer, Mum's eyes are drawn upwards. She points to a small golden figure entwined round the legs of a larger one. 'Look, Amelia,' she says. 'It's us. You were always clinging to me when you were little, hiding behind my legs, too shy to greet anyone, even family.'

Annie and Ben are already in The Oasis. Ben is making himself a coffee, while Annie sits at the table, engrossed in the pamphlet Eliza gave us last week.

'These booklets contain lists of sounds, words and phrases that you'll be recorded reading next Saturday,' Eliza explained then, passing the pamphlets around the circle. 'Your recordings will be uploaded to earpieces that will be given to your Partner. Wearing these earpieces will help you familiarise yourself with your Partner's consciousness. It's the first stage in your acclimatisation process. I recommend wearing the earpieces for short bursts during the first week. No more than twenty minutes of listening each day.'

Mum and I exchange quick hugs with Ben before she joins Annie at the table. She pulls out her notebook and begins flipping through the pages. I go to make her a coffee, then think better of it. She'll lecture anyone who will listen about there being no link between caffeine and Alzheimer's, only to blame the coffee when she becomes confused. 'Why did you let me drink this, Amelia?' she'll say. 'You know caffeine worsens my symptoms.'

I make myself a double espresso. Ben looks like he's had a restless night too; his eyes are bloodshot and weary. He watches Mum with a contemplative expression. She's holding her notebook close to her face – I suspect she's forgotten to put her contact lenses in.

Ben turns to me. 'I think you're remarkable for doing this,' he says. 'How old are you again? Twenty-three?'

I nod, and he exhales deeply. 'The possibility of Alzheimer's at your age. Not many people would take the chance.'

Annie is still focused on the pamphlet, her lips silently forming the words as she reads. 'What you're doing is just as brave,' I say. 'Your baby will be the first of its kind. I can't imagine how terrifying that must be.'

Ben nods. 'What's the alternative? At least this way our child gets a chance.'

Mum turns the page of her notebook, her brow furrowed in concentration.

'Is it difficult?' Ben asks.

I shrug. 'A lot of the time, it's easy to forget she's unwell. But then she has a bad day and it's like she's disappeared. Those days are hard. I'm not looking forward to the time when the bad days outnumber the good ones.' I down my espresso, the bitterness sharp on my tongue, and wipe my mouth with the back of my hand. The rehearsed line slips out smoothly. 'That's why we're here. Why I'm doing this. To make sure we never reach that point.'

We spend the morning in a recording booth. 'It's important that you enunciate clearly so our team can effectively transfer your speech onto the earpieces,' Eliza says. 'We want your words to be clear and distinct.'

I suggest that Mum be supervised to ensure she doesn't keep repeating the same words and phrases. Nathan accompanies her into the booth. When we reunite in The Oasis, she smiles. 'I rather enjoyed it,' she says. 'I felt like a radio presenter wearing those ridiculously large headphones.'

She swallows her medication and considers the selection of baked goods available for our morning snack. We chat with Jay and Noah as we eat our croissants. 'The earpieces are like hearing aids,' Noah says, adjusting his beanie. It's black today and, again, it matches his top. 'I looked them up online. Apparently, you can hardly tell when someone's wearing one.'

'I'm rather looking forward to having your thoughts in my head, Amelia,' Mum says through a mouthful of croissant. 'It will make a nice change from my own senseless ramblings.'

Our break ends, and we're divided into our roles. Mum and the other Transfers head to Room Two with Nathan. Annie, Jay, Lucas and I return to Room One. We take the same seats as before, leaving gaps between us. Eliza sits across from me. Her hair is down today, falling over her shoulders, a veil softening her edges.

She smiles. 'I want to begin by thanking the four of you for your incredible sacrifice. As Hosts of these revolutionary Merges, you are creating real hope for people who currently feel they have none. If we get this right, you won't only be saving your Partner, you'll be changing the lives of millions of desperate people.' She lets her words settle before her expression shifts. 'As with all experiments, there's a small chance the Merges will be unsuccessful. As I'm sure you know, over ninety-eight per cent of standard Merges are now completely successful, and those who are unfortunate enough to have a failed Merge tend to go on to live happy and healthy lives.'

I nod. I've spent a lot of time researching the Merges that went wrong. Most failures happened back when the standard Merge was still experimental. The research and video footage support what Eliza's saying: the Combines of the failed Merges did seem happy, but with an unfiltered, almost childlike happiness. Show them a balloon, and they'd laugh. Some seemed vacant, like Jonathan-Maria, cocooned in their own private world. They'd point at things that weren't there and giggle.

'Chances are,' Eliza continues, 'you have the same high probability of success as those undergoing the standard

Merge. You have been selected based on your compatibility scores, which makes a successful transfer extremely likely.' She rests her hands in her lap. 'Let me be clear. You are under no obligation to go through with this. If, at any point during your three-month Preparation Period, you decide you no longer want to proceed with the Merge, that's entirely acceptable.'

She pauses, scanning the room. 'What I'd love to do is properly learn why each of you is here. You gave us a brief introduction last week, but that was in front of the Transfers. This break-off group is your safe space. It's where you'll share the thoughts you don't want your Partners to hear, where you'll offload your doubts, anxieties, even resentment. No one enters the Preparation Period without these feelings. It's normal and healthy, and I encourage you to be open about how you feel. You've all signed the paperwork, so you understand that what is said in this room is strictly confidential. The more honest you are, the better we can help you prepare.' She looks around the circle. 'So, who would like to start us off?'

The four of us remain silent.

Then Lucas raises his hand.

Without Noah next to him, Lucas appears younger than before. His nose and cheeks are dotted with freckles, as if someone has flicked a paintbrush across his skin. His hair is an awkward length, requiring him to sweep it out of his eyes every few minutes. It reminds me of Albie when he was growing his hair out – Mum eventually became so frustrated by his constant fussing that she bought him an Alice band.

Lucas adjusts the collar of his polo shirt and returns Eliza's smile.

'Tell us why you're here, Lucas,' Eliza says. 'We know about Noah, but what we don't know is what led you to do this wonderful thing for your brother. Perhaps you could tell us more about how you came to be here today.'

Lucas's hand finds his fringe again. 'Noah's leukaemia is terminal,' he says, blinking to shift a stray strand. 'And I have the chance to save him. The doctors told us there's nothing more they can do, no options left, except this one. It was a no-brainer. Noah isn't just my brother. He's my best mate.'

Eliza smiles, and Annie does too, her hands gently resting on her stomach.

'How do your parents feel about you and Noah doing this?' Eliza asks.

'They're... conflicted,' Lucas says. 'It's difficult for them. They have different views from me and Noah. They always have.' He smiles faintly. 'You should have seen them the day the Merge was officially approved. They acted like it was the end of the world, like you'd have to be the devil to do it. And now here I am, their beloved son, the devil incarnate.'

I was with Albie the day the Merge received its first funding. He was lounging on the sofa, watching *Extinction*, fanning himself with a copy of the *Fortean Times*. On the screen, a polar bear was hunting for food, swimming so elegantly that I stood, transfixed. 'Why do you watch this, Albs? Doesn't it depress you?'

'Massively.' Albie shifted on the sofa, making room for me. I sat down, trying to ignore the polar bear's struggle by scrolling through my phone. The internet had exploded. I flicked through articles, refusing to believe what I was reading: Combine, the company behind the experiment causing worldwide outrage, was receiving billions in government funding. Winston and Adelaide, the two scientists everyone had written off as insane, were merging. Combining. Becoming one.

I passed my phone to Albie, too stunned to speak.

He glanced from the phone to me, and back again, frowning. It was a while before either of us spoke, and, when we did, all we could say was, *fuck*.

On the screen, the polar bear had succumbed to starvation.

'Were you anticipating such a negative reaction from your parents?' Eliza asks.

Lucas shrugs. 'I didn't really get why they acted so surprised. It had been, what, two years since the Merge was first trialled? Since Winston-Adelaide became Our Combine. Two years on and they were thriving, along with everyone else brave enough to sign up for the trials. I thought it was a good thing that they were opening it up to the whole of the UK. Noah thought so too. But my parents didn't see it that way. Dad called it immoral. We tried to argue that it was immoral *not* to be open to it, but he wouldn't listen. He said he thought he knew everything when he was young too, told us to give it twenty years and see how we felt.'

He pushes his fringe out of his eyes again. 'That's what gets me, his assumption that we've got twenty years left. He rolled his eyes when Mum cried over the tsunami in Spain, said she was being melodramatic. As long as we're okay, his family, then the world's okay in Dad's eyes. And we are okay. At least, we were that day. Noah was in remission, and it was before any of the non-Combine laws had been introduced. So, yeah, he didn't see the world burning as his problem to solve.'

Annie raises a tentative hand, and Lucas welcomes her question with a smile.

'I don't want to speak out of turn,' she says, instinctively returning her hand to her stomach. 'But, obviously, no one's ever merged with someone suffering from terminal cancer before, not that I know of anyway. Have you considered…

Have you thought about the potential implications of the Merge on you? On your health?'

'Have I considered that I might get cancer?'

She nods.

'Of course I have. I still want to do it. I'd take that chance a million times over to save Noah. I've spent years wishing I could do this – take the cancer from him. And now I can.'

Laurie

Amelia is sitting by herself in The Oasis. She's tucked away in the corner, sunk deep in one of the large, squishy chairs filled with tiny beads, the sort you can mould into different shapes. I'm standing close by, racking my brain for the name of these peculiar chairs, when Amelia spots me.

'Mum!' She pushes herself up from the comfy seat and envelops me in a tight hug as if we've not seen each other in months. 'How was your session?'

'Fine, fine,' I reply with a laugh, rubbing her back. She's far too thin, her spine prominent beneath my hand. 'How was yours?'

'Emotional,' she says, still clinging to me. 'Draining, actually.'

We pull apart, and she gently touches my face, resting her hand lightly on my cheek, the way I used to comfort her when she was little. 'What happened in your group?' she asks.

'I believe we're not allowed to talk about it,' I say. This rule is useful. It spares me the ordeal of recalling the session's details. It was mostly the angry young girl speaking. I jotted down bits and pieces. Enough, hopefully. I try to be selective with my notes. When there's too much scribbled on the page, the words are difficult to decipher.

'Sit down, Mum,' Amelia says, her voice gentle. 'I'll get you a green tea.'

'Thank you, sweetheart,' I say, though I can't understand why she thinks I'd want green tea. I settle into the low seat next to the one Amelia was using, open my notebook and begin to read.

TRANSFERS ONLY NOTES

Merge = very important. Big risk. Change the world.
Good thing to do!
Lara, 17 (see p10)
Struggles w/ addiction (started 13 at party, offered cocaine – hospitalised x5 – rehab x2 – heroin)
Who: Dad, Jay (see p9) Mum also volunteered but L more compatible with J.
L clean now, promises to stay clean. Doesn't need Merge to help her. Doesn't want to die. Doesn't always like J – annoys her – don't agree – how will she cope? Has offered to—

'Here you are, Mum.' Amelia reappears, holding a steaming mug and a plate with two cupcakes. I quickly close the notebook, smiling up at her.

'Thank you,' I say, and carefully adjust myself on the seat before taking the mug from her. The tea bag is still steeping, staining the water a murky green. I take a tentative sip and wince, then quickly set the mug on the floor, abandoning the grassy water. 'That's lovely,' I say. 'Just what I needed.'

Amelia sits beside me and passes me a cupcake, iced with the Combine mandala. I study the delicate pattern of the two brains before looking at her. 'How was your session?' I ask.

A flicker crosses Amelia's eyes. 'Emotional,' she says. 'Really quite draining.'

'You've already told me that, haven't you?'

She rests her hand on mine, and I sigh. We sit in silence for a while, Amelia absentmindedly picking at her nails, me staring at the closed notebook on my lap.

'Lara was talking in my session,' I say eventually. 'It's a difficult time for her, but I feel like I can help her somehow. I think I can reassure her.' I look at Amelia, so small in the large seat that it seems to swallow her. 'It's funny, this whole thing, isn't it?'

'How so?'

'Well, this girl needs convincing that she can't remain clean on her own, that if she's going to have a worthwhile future her father has to save her. It's so different to everything people are usually told. It's just... funny.'

I wait for Amelia to rationalise this for me, to laugh and tell me I'm ridiculous to think it's strange. I wait for her to roll her eyes and say, *It's the only way she'll be okay, Mum. Her dad wouldn't be doing this otherwise. They've exhausted all other options.* But she remains silent. She seeks the young girl out and watches her, as though she's sorry.

'Is that what they told her? That she needed to do this to get clean?'

'I can't remember specifically. But if my notes are any indication...'

Amelia eyes my closed notebook. 'How do you feel about having everyone over for dinner next week?' she says. 'I think it would be nice to get to know each other properly, outside of this place.'

'Really? It's not like you to want people over.'

'I think it's important. I'd like to get to know everyone better. What about inviting them over next Friday? For your birthday?'

'I'd be honoured.'

Amelia smiles, and I smile too. It's not the prospect of a birthday meal that excites me, but the thought of Amelia wanting to get to know new people. Her lack of interest in expanding her social circle, choosing instead to stay home with me, has been one of my biggest concerns regarding my dementia. Her being cooped up at home, caring for me once I'm no longer able to care for myself. I put my half-eaten cupcake down next to Amelia's. She's only taken a small bite of hers.

The film is shown to us in a large circular room. It feels like a planetarium. The chairs, slightly reclined, aren't in rows but curved into a horseshoe shape. The screen stretches along the walls and onto the ceiling.

'We'll soon be opening the cinema to the public.' Eliza paces slowly in front of the screen. She speaks loudly, as though addressing an audience far larger than the eight of us. 'We hope these films will inspire open-minded individuals such as yourselves to consider their role in sustaining our future. Fair warning, it's not especially pleasant viewing, but it's necessary. Vital, in fact. I hope that, for all of you here, the film instils in you a sense of honour and reminds you just how important your sacrifice is.'

The room goes dark. I blink at my notebook, straining to make out the faint blue lines on the pages. Amelia reaches for my arm. 'I'll remind you,' she whispers. 'We can take notes together once the film is finished.'

I nod, swallowing hard, refusing to let any tears spill. How pathetic to tear up just because the lights went out. But I rely on my notes. Without them, I'm utterly lost.

The film begins, and Amelia tightens her grip on my arm.

The opening shot is a sweeping bird's-eye view of London, revealing a panorama of skyscrapers and historic architecture gilded by the morning sun. The River Thames flows freely, its water level healthy, a vital artery winding through the city.

As the scene unfolds, a voiceover begins. 'London,' it intones, 'was once a vibrant metropolis, a dynamic hub of culture and commerce.'

We watch as happy people move among one another on streets that are busy but not crowded. Shops bustle with customers. Covent Garden brims with street performers, artists and applauding crowds. Tourists browse the produce at Borough Market, enjoying lively conversations with the vendors.

'Not long ago, Londoners lived in harmony with nature, enjoying green spaces and tranquil parks.'

The scene shifts to Richmond Park before the construction of those ghastly flats, erected without a thought for their design. Grey brick sores on the landscape. Children run through the grass, their laughter reverberating around the cinema. I smile, remembering Amelia splashing about in the fountain in Hyde Park, Mitchell laughing as she squealed with delight at getting soaked.

The cheerful images fade, and the upbeat music is replaced by a sombre string-heavy soundtrack. I'm reminded of Elgar, or Walton maybe. 'In a few short years,' the voiceover continues, 'the world we once knew has crumbled under the weight of our own excess and neglect.'

We're shown shots of London today: tired crowds moving slowly in packs, unable to pass one another. Shops boarded up, those still open sporting patched and broken windows. Bloodied security guards huddled outside.

'The aftermath of last winter's looting serves as a grim reminder of the lengths to which desperate individuals have been forced to go to secure essential items. It is not the fault of any single person, but rather the consequence of our collective failure to confront the looming threats.'

A montage of newsclips plays. We watch scenes from our overstretched hospitals, listen as nurses and doctors break down in tears. 'The National Health Service,' the voiceover declares, 'once a beacon of healthcare excellence, now struggling to cope with the relentless pressures of a world in crisis.'

Then comes a harrowing montage of disasters from around the world. The Netherlands in the wake of the floods: a woman weeps as she wades through her front room, a crying toddler clinging to her hip, furniture floating around her. The droughts in Somalia, Sudan and Yemen flash by – shots of arid landscapes, parched fields and desperate people searching for water. We see the wildfires that scorched through Australia, the US and southern Europe. The mass migrations of Kiribati and Tuvalu, and the subsequent bloody conflict. Crop failures in India. The relentless spread of disease.

I can't bear it any longer. I close my eyes. I'd forgotten the extent of the horrors that have filled these past years. How many years has it been? When did it all begin? Was Mitchell still here when the world started to crumble, or did he escape before then?

I open my eyes. On the screen a familiar-looking man dressed in a suit – the prime minister, I presume – stands solemnly in front of 10 Downing Street. 'Our world is facing an unprecedented challenge, a crisis that threatens not only our environment but the very fabric of our society and economy.'

Newspaper headlines plaster the screen, variations of the same urgent messages.

The screen fades to white.

A shot of an empty chair slowly comes into focus. Footsteps echo softly. A woman wearing a forest-green robe, her hair neatly styled in a bun, enters the frame. She sits and smiles at someone just out of view.

When she speaks, her voice is slow. Careful. As though she's weighing each word. 'For years,' she begins, 'we were warned about the repercussions of our growing population.

We knew, with absolute certainty, that our resources were finite, and dwindling rapidly, that our immediate future was not guaranteed.'

An image of the woman, visibly younger and wearing a lab coat, appears on her left. On her right, a young man in a matching coat materialises. 'Having dedicated our lives to environmental research and activism, we – Winston and Adelaide – began working with politicians to push for stronger climate policies. While it initially seemed that we were being listened to, we soon found ourselves frustrated by the lack of urgency among decision-makers.'

The screen fills once again with shots of wildfires, floods and protests. A furious crowd, a seething mass of environmental activists.

Amelia grips my hand tightly. She's searching for him, just as I am.

'This is what it took,' the woman says, 'what it came to. The world reached breaking point before we were finally heard.' The images fade. 'But it was too late. The crisis had gone too far for the strategies we'd hoped would be successful. We had to rethink our approach, not only to environmental protection, but also to the very essence of what it means to be human.'

The woman smiles, and the upbeat music from the beginning of the film resumes. 'With the support of visionary leaders and the dedication of countless scientists and activists, we' – she gestures to the images of her younger self and the young man – 'founded Combine, a company committed to pushing the boundaries of possibility in the pursuit of restoring our climate. Through tireless research and radical advancements, we discovered a way to merge our minds and bodies, amplifying our strengths and surpassing the limitations of individuality. We chose to be the first to put our theory to the test and merge, to exist in one body and halve our environmental footprint.'

The images fade, leaving only the woman in the chair.

Not a woman, I now remember. A Combine.

Two people in one.

Winston and Adelaide.

Our Combine.

'But our journey is far from over. The Merge is not just about combining two individuals. It is about the merging of humanity towards a shared destiny. It's about recognising that our differences are our greatest strength and that, together, we have the power to heal our planet.' They twist in the chair and point to the tattoo on their neck. 'Merge and pave the way to a brighter future.'

Winston-Adelaide fades, and an array of Combines pop up across the screen, each dressed in the same forest-green robe. One by one, they speak of their lives before the Merge. We listen to tales of exhaustion, ill health and overwhelming guilt. They speak of financial struggles and appalling living conditions. Then the narrative shifts. They begin speaking of their current lives, how much happier they are, how much stronger, more fulfilled. Their faces brighten as they describe the financial relief provided by tax breaks, the housing generously gifted to them by Combine. They tell us about their improved job opportunities, their greater societal influence, their vastly increased quality of life.

One by one, the happy faces fade from the screen, until only a swirling grey background remains. Then Winston-Adelaide reappears, smiling in their green robe.

'Why not try it?' they say.

The screen fades to black.

Laurie

I'm wearing the earpieces that contain Amelia's voice. I like to wear them when she's out, to have her keep me company when I'm alone. She worries I'll become dependent on the recordings for comfort, but I won't. I'm careful. I make a conscious effort to remove the earpieces every so often, to embrace moments of silence.

What Amelia talks about in the recordings is often dull. I tend not to pay too much attention to the words, just letting the cadence of her voice quieten my mind. Sometimes I catch myself speaking aloud, replying to her, expecting a response. It makes me laugh when I remember she's not really there.

Amelia chats away as I sort out the apartment. *What a lovely day. Perfect picnic weather. We could go to the park and enjoy the sun. Throw a frisbee or play football.* Her voice is welcome background noise as I organise the drawers and tidy up the bookshelves. Everything gets in such a muddle these days. One moment the apartment is clean and tidy, everything in its place, and the next it's as though someone's ransacked every room. Invariably, I am that 'someone'. I'll be partway through a task, remember something I forgot to do earlier and rush to complete it, leaving a trail of misplaced items in my wake.

Just now, for instance, I was flipping through a book when I remembered the art supplies left out on the dining room table. I started clearing them away and accidentally knocked over a vase of flowers, sending water and petals cascading over my half-finished painting of the roses, turning it into a soggy mess of colours.

I take a moment to collect myself. It's only a bit of water. Nothing broken. Nothing worth getting upset about. I reach for the fallen vase, but my elbow nudges a tray of paintbrushes, sending them clattering to the floor. I close my eyes, a lump forming in my throat. Everything I touch seems to lead to chaos.

All the while, Amelia's voice continues. *I think I'd like to plant vegetables and contribute to a more self-sufficient lifestyle. We could save money and connect with nature.*

I open my eyes, place the vase back on the table, and try to salvage what I can of the roses. Once everything is cleared up, I carry the bag of art supplies to my room. I used to have a studio, a little annexe in the garden, where I'd retreat after work. Mitchell would deliver me cups of tea, even dinner on nights when I became too immersed in my painting to stop. 'Just a bite,' he'd say. 'A nibble.' I'd begrudgingly comply, and we'd laugh as he teased me for being as stubborn as a toddler.

Now, I make do with painting at the dining table, clearing away my work between meals. Sometimes I forget, and Amelia gets cross. 'This place is small enough without all your clutter.'

As I pass her room, I notice something of mine on her desk. My notebook, open on a double page. I hover in the doorway, hesitant to intrude. I don't like to enter Amelia's space when she's not around. She's a grown woman, forced to live with her mother in a cramped flat, and I strive to make that as easy as possible for her by keeping my nose out of her business.

I should probably start eating healthier. It's so difficult though. How are you supposed to resist all these tempting snacks?

I put down the bag of art supplies and remove the earpieces.

Did I give Amelia my notebook to help me write up something about the sessions? Or has she taken it without permission? I'm sure I've told her I'd prefer she not read my notes, at least not without me there. I enter her room. Her bed is made, the covers pulled tight, pillows perfectly plump and carefully placed. No matter the state of the apartment, Amelia's bedroom remains immaculate. She inherited Mitchell's meticulousness. He was forever straightening the sofa cushions, unable to abide them being askew. We'd be chatting, and I'd notice his eyes flitting towards the sofa. 'Go on,' I'd say. 'Sort it out so you can stop worrying and concentrate on me.' When Mitchell passed, I tried my best to keep the house up to his standards, but it soon fell into disarray.

I sit at Amelia's desk. It's not unusual for me to be here. I'm familiar with the view of her incredibly large monitor and the neatly stacked hard drives, each labelled with a different letter of the alphabet. She has backups of backups. Not one for risks, is my daughter.

I often join Amelia at her desk when she's editing. I like to watch as she drags clips onto the timeline and the video starts to take shape. 'That's a great shot,' she'll say on the rare occasion I've managed to film something worthy of inclusion in the final product. 'You're getting good at this, Mum.'

Amelia 'hired' me to assist on her shoots after the school made me redundant. At first, I didn't do much filming. Amelia set everything up, and I stood nervously behind the camera, praying it was doing what it was supposed to. But over time, I've grown more confident.

Now, I can set up the tripod myself. I enjoy it. I take time to ensure it's at precisely the right height, perfectly level, and in exactly the right position for the shot we need. I like twisting the camera onto the tripod's attachment, securing it tightly before adjusting it and setting it in place.

I check behind me, just in case Amelia has returned. It feels wrong to be in her room without her, reading this notebook, even though it belongs to me.

The handwriting on the page isn't mine but Amelia's. I must have asked her to help me make sense of something, but I can't recall what.

I begin reading, using my finger to track the words.

Propaganda film today – discomforting parallels between the film's rhetoric and historical propaganda – authenticity of film's footage? Emotional manipulation? Mum shut eyes during most intense parts of film. Visibly distressed. Varied reactions among Participants. Some visibly shaken, others—

The doorbell rings.

I jump, quickly closing the notebook.

It's not Amelia at the door, but Mary. She's standing there, holding a large bouquet of sunflowers – Mitchell's favourite – her hood pulled up against the rain. I peer up at the dark sky. I could have sworn it was nice out. Blue skies and sunshine. Perfect weather for a picnic.

'Are you okay, Lor?' Mary asks, stepping inside and removing her wet coat. She wipes her boots on the doormat, darkening it with streaks of mud.

I take her coat and hang it on one of the hooks just inside the front door. It drips onto Amelia's denim jacket. We used to have a boot room. Amelia would tuck her red wellingtons between mine and Mitchell's. 'A family of wellies,' she'd say.

I'm unsure if I was expecting Mary's arrival or if this is a spontaneous visit. I've no memory of her mentioning she'd be stopping by. 'You needn't have brought me these,' I say, taking the sunflowers from her. Rain slides down the protective cellophane and runs inside my sleeve. 'Since when do we give each other flowers? Come on inside, you're soaking. I'll make you a nice cup of tea.'

I go to the lounge to fetch the vase from the mantelpiece. I'll chuck the roses. They're nearing the end of their life. But the vase isn't there. I frown at the empty space where the roses should be. I go back to the hallway to tell Mary that the vase has disappeared and find her still standing on the doormat, her boots still on. 'What is it?' I say. 'What's wrong?'

'Is Amelia home?'

'No. She's working. What is it, Mary? Has something happened?'

Mary addresses the flowers in my hands. 'It's July the twelfth,' she says quietly. 'I've been at the park all morning. I've been calling you, but you didn't answer.'

I pat my empty trouser pockets. 'I haven't got my phone on me. I've probably left it in the lounge or…' I frown. 'Have I forgotten something?'

The lack of colour in Mary's face provides the answer. I've forgotten something big. Something she'd never expect me to forget.

'It's the anniversary of Mitchell's death, Lor,' she says. 'It's ten years today.'

I shake my head. I couldn't have forgotten Mitchell's anniversary. I've been dreading it for weeks. Amelia has caught me more than once, counting down the days on the calendar, bracing myself for its arrival.

Mary finally removes her boots.

'You're wrong,' I say. 'You've got the wrong day. It's not…' I walk into the kitchen and dump the sunflowers on the counter. I go to the calendar and run my finger slowly along the dates, trying to remember what day Mary said it was. My finger stops on the square marked with Mitchell's name.

July twelfth.

'It's today?'

She nods.

I put my hand to my mouth. 'What's wrong with me?'

'Oh, Lor.'

'I'm going mad, Mary.'

'No, you're not. You're just confused, Lor.'

'I've never forgotten something this important before. I know what they say about how it progresses, but I'm fine otherwise. I'm...' I trail off, looking around the kitchen. Plates are piled high, and countless mugs of cold tea clutter the counters – cups I've forgotten to finish. Notebooks of various sizes are stacked on the kitchen table. One lies open, its pages covered in blue ink. Many of the cupboards hang open, displaying a jumble of jars, tins and packets, the disorganised nature of which would have caused Mitchell to have an aneurysm. Mitchell. My darling Mitchell.

How could I forget?

I set about shutting the cupboards, slamming the doors closed. They're covered in sticky notes, each one labelling what's inside. I'd started using them after spending too much time taking everything out, hunting for something we didn't have. Tears spill before I can stop them. I rip off the sticky notes, scrunching them into a tight ball.

What have I become?

How have I let things get so out of hand?

How long have I been like—

Mary holds me to her, cradling the back of my head. She keeps hold until the tears slow, then uses her sleeve to wipe them away. 'Have you taken your medicine?'

I check the pill box and find that this morning's tablets

remain untouched. Mary pours me a glass of water, and I swallow the pills. 'Why don't I make us some lunch,' she suggests. 'We can have a quick tidy, then we'll head to the park and visit that dear husband of yours.'

The rain has stopped by the time we reach the park, the familiar cobblestone path washed clean. The sun has broken through the grey clouds. 'See, Lor,' Mary says, spreading a blanket over Mitchell's bench. 'You always bring the sunshine with you.'

'Mitch used to call me his sunshine,' I say. 'He said his world revolved around me.'

'I know he did.' She passes me the flask of tea and carefully places two china cups on the arm of the bench. 'I'll be over by the pond,' she says, giving my shoulder a squeeze before walking away. 'You two have a good catch-up.'

I pour Mitchell his cup of tea first and place it beside me on the bench. The engraved brass plaque on the backrest catches my eye: *Mitchell Jonathan Anderson. A cherished husband, father, brother and friend whose heart was devoted to his wife Laurie and daughter Amelia.* The inscription has always made me feel guilty, what it omitted.

Who it omitted.

I push the guilt aside and promise myself I'll come and give the plaque a much-needed polish. Then I pour my own cup of tea and take a sip. 'Proper builder's tea,' I tell him. 'Just how we like it.'

Mitchell and I had a routine. Every evening before bed we'd sit together on the sofa and enjoy a cuppa. He'd put the kettle on, drown the tea bags and set the timer. I'd get out the biscuit tin and bring it to the conservatory. We'd sit together, chatting as our tea brewed for exactly four minutes. I'd carry the steaming mugs from the kitchen, and we'd talk about our days, sipping contentedly, squeezed close on a single cushion, sharing a triangle of shortbread.

We met in a café in Islington. The walls were decorated with the work of local artists, a painting or two of mine among them. In the centre of the café stood a long table with benches on either side, dubbed the 'social table'. It was where I liked to sit, nestled in the heart of the activity. I rarely joined in the conversations, but I listened as I sketched.

The day I met Mitchell, we were sitting on opposite sides of the table, he engrossed in an old Agatha Christie – *A Murder is Announced* – and me sketching him as he turned the pages. When he stood to leave, tucking his book into his bag, he asked to see the drawing.

I flushed. 'Was I that obvious?'

He made to lie, to spare me the embarrassment, but then decided on honesty – a trait he maintained for all our years together. 'You were as conspicuous as a peacock at a camouflage convention,' he said with a laugh. 'What was it you were having trouble with? You kept rubbing something out and sighing. It was disconcerting. I tried my best to stay still for you.'

'Your mouth,' I said. 'I'm not good at mouths.'

Our first date was a picnic beneath an umbrella. We popped a bottle of prosecco, and he rested his lips against mine so gently that I ached with desire.

What I wouldn't give to kiss him one last time.

I look at Mitchell's teacup beside me. 'Do you know what we're doing, Mitch? Have you been watching us? I feel you next to me sometimes.' I take another sip of tea, waiting for his response. I'll feel it, like I always do, that warmth spreading through my chest. 'I won't be going through with it, Mitch. Don't you worry about that. It's just... you know how Amelia is, how she's been since you left. She blames herself, you know, for you not being here. I know that's not nice to hear, but it's true. I'm sure of it. She spends so many hours holed up in her room. She never used to hide away, did she? Not when you were here.'

I sit a while, listening to the birds. Mitchell would have known exactly what birds they were; he could identify them from their very first notes.

I clear my throat. 'Today, for the first time, I forgot about you, Mitch. I'm so sorry. It wasn't for long and I'm sure I would've remembered eventually, even without Mary turning up to remind me. But the point is, I forgot.'

I take a deep breath. 'It made me think. What if Amelia isn't crazy when she says that merging is the right thing to do? Maybe blending my mind with hers really would be the lesser of two evils. At least that way I'll never forget you. What do you think? Is fusing my mind with hers better than losing it altogether?'

Amelia

Everyone is over to celebrate Mum's birthday. She's noticeably happier now that our guests have arrived. It's a relief to see her smiling. I was worried she wouldn't snap out of her bad mood and that this evening would turn unbearably awkward.

This morning, I woke to find her standing over me, notebook in hand. 'It's not right,' she said. 'This "merging" isn't ethical. You should live in the body you're born in and leave well enough alone.'

I tried to hide under the duvet, but she lifted it off me. 'I'm serious, Amelia. I've been reading my notes and it's all so incredibly sad. These people need help. That poor girl battling addiction. She needs a rehabilitation centre, not to blend her mind with someone else. And what about us, Amelia? Why must we be the first? Why can't we let someone else with Alzheimer's do this ghastly experiment and see how they get on? Someone who is absolutely certain this is what they want?'

I sat up, checking the time. It was barely five. 'I'm not forcing you to do this, Mum,' I said, my voice thick with sleep. 'I'm just asking you to try. Keep going with the Preparation Period and see how you feel at the end.'

'My mind won't be changed.'

'That's fine. Just don't quit before you know for sure.'

She's been furious with me all day, storming around the house and slamming doors. She only calms down when she forgets. Then she reads her notebook again, and the cycle repeats.

I was tempted to cancel the dinner party, but now that everyone's here, I'm glad I didn't. Mum's all smiles, her earlier irritation forgotten, as though she hasn't spent the day angered by the very people surrounding her, furious about their decision to merge.

We've somehow managed to squeeze all eight of us round the table, shifting on stools and wedging ourselves into corners with elbows pressed close to our sides. Mary couldn't come because she 'wasn't feeling well'. I know the real reason is her unease at the idea of spending an evening with people on the verge of merging. In a way, it's a relief she didn't come; we're cramped as it is, and her pointed glances wouldn't have helped Mum's mood.

A birthday banner is taped to the kitchen wall, covering the worst of the cracked paintwork. We keep talking about repairing and repainting the wall, but we can't bring ourselves to do it. Repainting would make the apartment ours, and we're not ready for that. We never will be.

Our home, draped in wisteria, was loved, and well lived in. 'A fairy's house,' Dad used to say. 'A house of magic and spells.' And I believed him. I believed I lived in a magical house because my parents made it feel that way.

'They'll have to carry me out,' Mum said the day she received her eviction notice. 'I'm not leaving, Amelia. They can't make me leave.'

The change came overnight. An announcement: all non-Combines residing in private housing would be required to pay a new tax. The funds collected from this tax would be allocated to providing enhanced resources and support for the Combine community, who play an integral role in our collective progress and prosperity.

When the letter arrived, we read it together. The tax was in no way proportionate to Mum's meagre income. 'They've made a mistake,' I said. 'They've sent the letter to the wrong address.'

A couple of months passed before the armed officers turned up and forcibly escorted Mum from our home, their grip leaving dark bruises on her wrists. She was dragged from her three-bedroom fairy cottage, with Dad's lovingly tended garden and the olive tree planted in his memory, into one of the grey stone apartment blocks, crammed with other non-Combines who could no longer afford their homes.

Mum managed to get an apartment before the block filled up, which it soon did. There was no affordable accommodation left, but that didn't stop the evictions. The houses stood empty. Furnished. Waiting. To live in one, all you had to do was merge. And people did. Hundreds of thousands signed up for the privilege of getting their homes back.

Annie stands, holding a glass of alcohol-free champagne. I'm filming her, and the shot is beautiful, the brass lamp behind her bathing her in a warm orange glow. Mum spent ages fiddling with the lights before everyone arrived, moving lamps, dimming and brightening bulbs. She wanted to create the perfect ambience.

'To Lor!' Annie announces, lifting her glass.

'To Lor,' everyone echoes.

They clink their glasses together. I don't know if it's the lighting, the champagne flutes, or simply the joy of everyone coming together to celebrate Mum, but the moment feels perfect.

'And to Noah,' Jay says, raising his glass for a second toast. I shift the camera to focus on him. 'He'll be missed tonight, but we look forward to seeing him tomorrow.'

'To Noah,' we chorus.

'Thanks, Jay,' Lucas says. 'He was really sad to miss out.'

'He needs his rest,' Jay says. 'The sessions are pretty intense. What are we, three weeks in? I'm already wiped out. I can't imagine how tiring it must be for him.'

There's a round of 'Happy Birthday'. Mum notices the camera on her and takes a self-conscious sip of her drink. She used to bask in the glow of being the centre of attention. Now, she fears the gaze of others, convinced they see her for all the wrong reasons. 'Thank you,' she says, pressing the flute to her flushed cheek.

Lara drains her glass and looks around for a refill. I was worried about having alcohol available tonight, but Jay insisted it was fine: Lara would stick to the alcohol-free options. 'She's underage as it is,' he said. 'And she'd hate to be the reason no one else is drinking. Besides, she won't be the only one. Annie's not going to be having any alcohol, and Lucas is only fifteen.' The fact that Lara's champagne is alcohol free doesn't seem to have dampened her enthusiasm. She reaches over the bowl of crisps to refill her glass.

Albie catches my eye, his glass still raised, and winks at the camera.

We haven't spoken since we fucked in his kitchen.

Mum invited him without telling me. 'Surprise,' he said when I opened the door. He kissed me stiffly on the cheek. 'Lor thought it would be nice for me to meet everyone, and I didn't have the heart to say no.'

'Tonight isn't about your views on my Merge,' I said, letting him into the apartment. He waved at Mum, who was busy perfecting the lighting as we passed the lounge. 'This isn't about your view on what I, or any of these people, are doing. This is about Mum and her birthday.'

'It'll be her last birthday,' he said. 'Have you considered that?'

'I'm serious, Albie. Drop it. Just for tonight.'

Back at the table, Mum's steering the conversation in a new direction. 'That's a beautiful ring, Annie. Forgive me if I've already asked, but when are you getting married?'

'You're still having a wedding?' Lara says, raising an eyebrow. 'Don't people going through with the Merge just have Commitment Ceremonies now?'

'We're still not sure what we're going to do.' Annie stands and moves to the counter, waving at the camera as she passes. I've cooked, but she's going to do the serving. It was a condition of her attending. 'You and Laurie are hosts,' she said. 'So Ben and I will do everything else. You must relax and enjoy the night after putting so much effort into the food.'

'We've got a date for the wedding,' she says, picking up the carving knife. 'It's meant to be happening next month, but it seems a bit redundant now.'

'Yeah,' Ben says. 'We booked the venue long before the bump came along.'

'It would still be a lovely day,' Mum says. 'A celebration of your love before your lives change forever.'

Annie lifts the tin foil from the roast chicken. 'That's true,' she says. 'It might be nice to celebrate us while we are still us.'

Jay, seated across from Albie, nods. 'I'm with Lor. Best day of my life, marrying Kath.'

Albie is quiet, his fingers absently tracing the edge of his glass.

Ben moves to join Annie at the counter. 'I'm not convinced there's much point in having a wedding these days.' He starts transferring roasted vegetables onto the plates. 'Lara's right, most people are opting for Commitment Ceremonies now. It's essentially the same thing, isn't it? Everyone comes together to celebrate you before you make the ultimate commitment to each other. Marriage hardly seems worth celebrating anymore.'

Mum's watching Albie, his fingers still tracing the glass's rim. She knows, like I do, what he's thinking about: me, us – the wedding he wants and knows he'll never have if I go through with this.

'Why don't you have a Commitment Ceremony, then?' Jay suggests. 'Kath is keen for me and Lara to have one. If an empty support circle is what you're worrying about, Ben, we can all be there to fill up seats.'

Ben chuckles. 'Kind of you, mate.'

Annie pauses mid-carve, raising her eyebrows at Jay. 'You're having a Ceremony?'

'No,' Lara says. 'We're not.'

'Kath wants us to. She wants the whole family there to celebrate us,' Jay says, grabbing a handful of crisps from the bowl. 'Lara isn't so keen.'

'It's gross,' Lara says flatly. 'I'm not doing it.'

'Noah and I are Committing,' Lucas says. 'I'm really looking forward to it. Ellie went to a Ceremony last year and said it was really special. Merging is a big deal. It should be properly celebrated.'

'Maybe we should, Annie,' Ben says. 'It might be nice.'

'I don't know.' Annie frowns, glancing between me and Mum. 'What about you two? Are you having a Ceremony?'

I look at Mum. Even though we've filmed lots of Ceremonies together, we've never discussed having one of our own. 'I don't know. Do you want to, Mum?'

Mum shakes her head with a small smile. 'All I want is chicken.'

Ben laughs. 'Hurry up, Annie. The birthday girl's hungry.'

There's a sparkle in Mum's eyes. It's been years since she hosted a party, since she's been surrounded by friends in her own home. Hosting has always been something she loved, something she insisted on. 'Why don't you have some friends over?' she'd ask whenever I was home doing nothing in the evenings. 'A house only becomes a home once you open the doors to others, Amelia.'

I'm not sure what made her stop having people over. I don't know whether it's because of the Alzheimer's diagnosis, the apartment or me being at home. Perhaps it's a combination of all three.

'My god, ladies,' Annie says, taking a seat at the table. 'This looks so delicious.'

'It really does,' Jay agrees, rubbing his hands together.

'It's all Amelia,' Mum says. 'She wouldn't let me lift a finger.'

I put the camera down and pick up my cutlery, gesturing for everyone to do the same. 'Thank you,' I say. 'Tuck in.'

We soon get through the two bottles of Champagne and are on to the pinot grigio. Annie keeps topping up our glasses. 'I'm living vicariously through you,' she insists whenever we protest. I relax back in my chair, allowing the tipsy feeling to wash over me. Lucas, who I doubt has much experience with alcohol, is slumped in the seat next to me, typing a long message on his phone.

'You could have brought Ellie along with you tonight,' I say. 'It would be lovely to meet her.'

Lucas sits up straighter, lighting up at the mention of Ellie's name. 'Want to see a picture of her?'

'Of course.'

He passes me his phone. His background is of Ellie cuddling a ginger cat. She's so young, with blond hair, a moon-shaped face and deep dimples. In the photo she wears glasses with clear frames, her smile bright and colourful with alternating pink and blue bands on her braces. 'She's beautiful, Lucas.'

He nods, glancing at his phone, anticipating Ellie's reply. I smile, remembering the early days of my relationship with Albie, the thrill of seeing his name light up my screen. 'How does she feel about you doing this?' I ask, handing his phone back.

'She's a bit nervous about it,' he says. 'But she supports me... She loves Noah, too.' He finishes the small amount of wine left in his glass. 'If you came to my apartment and saw what Noah's like tonight...' He swallows, his face reddening. 'He has these really low periods where no one can get through to him.'

'Lucas, I'm so sorry.'

'It's okay. I'm used to it.' He tries a smile. 'I'll be able to stop it, and that's what matters. He won't have to feel these things for much longer.' He nods across the table to Albie, who's chatting with Ben. 'Albie seems really nice. Are you guys feeling okay about staying together through all of this? I know everyone says it's difficult, but Ellie and I are determined to give it a good go.'

I look at Albie, his easy laughter. 'We're... It's hard to say.' I watch as he chats, his smile convincing. He looks like he genuinely wants to be here. Lucas gets a message from Ellie and starts typing a reply, his thumbs moving quickly.

'Amelia?'

I turn to Mum.

'What's wrong with you and Albie?'

I smile. 'Nothing, Mum. We're fine.'

'You're not.' She scoots her chair closer to mine. 'He's been watching you all evening. And you're not sitting together. You've hardly spoken. I heard what you just said to that boy. What's going on? Have you had a falling-out?'

Albie and I agreed not to tell Mum about our relationship ending. She's already unsure about merging, and even Albie agreed that his feelings shouldn't influence her decision. 'Amelia,' Mum says again. She waits until I'm fully focused on her. 'I know how worried you are about me. And I adore you for caring so much. But I can see how much this is affecting you. You're hardly eating, and you're spending all your days cooped up in your room. I hear you talking to yourself, and you never sound happy. You haven't been happy since I was diagnosed. I know it's hard, Amelia. But it's life. And *my* life at that. It's not yours to fix.'

I frown. 'You hear me talking to myself? When?'

'Whenever I pass your room. I don't mean to eavesdrop, Amelia, but this flat is so small. You always sound so stressed, so serious. What is it you're doing in there?'

Across the table, Albie's still talking to Ben, the two of them laughing easily as though they've known each other for years.

'What is it, Amelia? You're acting so strangely.'

'I'm sorry, Mum. It's just – a lot – having everyone over. Having Albie here, meeting...' My gaze lingers on him a moment longer before shifting back to her. 'It's two worlds colliding. It's overwhelming.'

'This is what I worry about, Amelia. This merging is going to change everything. And not for the better.' Her eyes search mine. 'It's already started. You're clearly uncomfortable.'

'I'm not uncomfortable, Mum.'

'I'm not buying—'

I shove my chair back and move to join Annie at the counter. Mum calls after me, her voice laced with frustration and concern. 'I can see how much this is affecting you. You think I don't notice, but I do.'

I busy myself with loading the dishwasher, my hands trembling. Annie watches. She bends slightly, her shoulder brushing mine as she whispers. 'Are you okay?'

I nod, forcing a smile as I stack the plates.

Then Albie laughs. That familiar sound, like rolling thunder. The walls of the flat close in, confining me, accusing me.

He laughs again.

I close my eyes. What was once my favourite sound now taunts me, reminds me of everything that's slipping away.

'Amelia,' Mum calls softly, but I don't turn round. I open my eyes, focusing on the task at hand, trying to hold back the tears that threaten to spill. I can feel Mum's gaze. Her plea for honesty, for connection.

'Amelia,' she calls again, her voice softer, almost breaking. 'Please, talk to me.'

'Later, Mum,' I whisper, barely audible. 'Not now.'

Amelia

Mum was diagnosed with Alzheimer's three years ago. The news came as most life-changing news does: quietly, on an ordinary day.

Albie and I were sitting on the tiny balcony of our flat, our legs up, our knees tucked under our chins. It was late September, and so hot that we had sodden flannels draped round our necks.

We'd recently moved in together. We'd done well to get an apartment; Albie's friend had been accepted for a Merge and gave him the heads-up before moving out. 'It's pretty fucking depressing,' he'd said, 'but it's there if you want it. Furnished and all.'

The flat was small and plain, a boxy living space with beige walls that always smelled faintly of damp, no matter how many times we aired it out.

Albie was telling me about the march he'd been on the day before. 'There were thousands of us,' he said, his words quick. 'It feels like everyone's getting behind the movement, like Combine will actually be stopped.' He pulled a pack of Pall Malls from his pocket and lit one. 'I'm not kidding,' he said, the smoke billowing from his mouth. 'It really did feel different this time.'

I never joined Albie on the marches, relying instead on his recounts to keep me informed. I supported the Anti-Merge movement in other ways: boycotting companies aligned with Combine, handing out pamphlets warning of the dangers of merging, volunteering at the local food bank to help those resisting, even when they couldn't afford to. Albie never pressured me to attend the rallies. He understood why I opted to stay home.

Mum had always panicked about me going on marches with Dad, but he took me along every chance he got. He insisted I be exposed to the truth. 'Knowledge without action,' he would say, 'is meaningless.'

I'd never understood Mum's fear. The marches were always peaceful, the protestors wanting only to raise awareness about various environmental threats. There was never any violence, despite the massive crowds. Often there was so little to do I became bored. I'd experiment with Dad's DSLR, spending hours with my face scrunched up in concentration, my eye pressed to the viewfinder, taking photos of the activists surrounding us.

'You're really talented, Mills,' Dad would say after taking the opportunity to look properly through my photos, something he always made time for. 'These are powerful images. Really, they are.'

I was supposed to be with him the day he died. He waited for me to get ready, but I refused to leave the house. I was upset because he'd broken his promise to take me to the cinema the night before. Such a stupid thing to be upset about, but I was.

I was fourteen, desperate to do the things my friends did on Friday nights and weekends. I vented my frustration at him, said I hated him for being so boring and spending his weekends marching. It didn't occur to me then that he was trying to make the world a better place for me, for all of us.

Dad didn't get cross when I shouted at him. He didn't send me to my room or ground me. He apologised, told me he was exhausted from work and promised to make it up to me; we'd go to the cinema after the march. But the offer wasn't good enough. I wanted him to know how betrayed I felt, so I made him go alone.

The march was infiltrated by counter-protestors. The heat of that summer had fanned the flames of societal anger, bringing rioters out in force, attacking anyone who opposed their worldview. We don't know what happened to Dad, why he was one of the few who didn't come home that day. 'He was protecting others,' Mum always says. 'Making sure they got out alive.' But there's no evidence of that.

I browsed the newspaper while Albie finished his cigarette. He listened, frowning, as I read aloud an article about the unprecedented rise in the numbers of people taking compatibility tests. When I handed him the paper, he took his turn reading aloud to me. He was halfway through an article about desert sand rapidly disappearing in the Middle East when my phone rang.

'Hello, Amelia.' Mum sounded strange, as though she had something caught in her throat. 'Where are you?'

'At the flat. Why? Are you okay, Mum?'

'Are you able to speak?'

Albie was silent, watching me curiously. I went into the lounge. 'What's going on? Are you okay? Has something—'

It hit me as soon as I asked.

I closed my eyes, pressing my fist into my forehead. How had I forgotten about her appointment? She'd been worrying about it for weeks, fretting over her tests and how they'd gone. 'I couldn't remember the words, Amelia,' she'd said, over and over in the days after. 'I kept muddling them up and missing them out.' Each time, I'd told her to stop worrying. 'If someone told me a list of words and made me wait five minutes before repeating them, I'd forget some, too. Everyone would, Mum. It doesn't mean anything.'

'What did the doctor say?' I opened my eyes, aware of how tightly I was holding the phone.

'Dementia,' Mum said. Just like that.

I froze in the middle of the lounge, my throat tight and dry.

'I suspected,' she said, no longer fighting back her tears. 'It's what I've been saying. I've been feeling so funny. I've been so... The other day I completely lost my bearings. I drove for hours trying to get back home.'

'Mum,' I finally whispered. 'How can you have dementia? You're not old enough.'

'Young onset Alzheimer's.' She managed a little laugh through her tears. 'And thank you for calling me young, darling, but I'm almost sixty-two. I'm only a few years away from it being regular Alzheimer's.'

'But you're fine, Mum. I don't understand... How can—'

'I'm not fine, Amelia.'

The way she said it splintered something inside me. I could feel the slow fracture, the sharp ache spreading through my chest. I shook my head, pinching the inside of my arm until it stung. 'Let's get a second opinion, Mum. How can they...'

'It is dementia, Amelia. I know it's dementia. I knew before they told me. I don't need a second opinion.'

Albie helped me shove my things into a suitcase. 'How long will you be gone?' he asked, carrying over an armful of underwear.

'I don't know.'

He nodded, dumped the underwear into the case and returned to the chest of drawers. 'I want to come with you.'

'Mum won't want that. I have to spend some time with her, just us two.'

He rummaged through the sock drawer, hunting for pairs. 'I'll come with you to the station, make sure you get on the tube.'

At the station, Albie kissed me. 'Promise you won't stay there forever,' he said.

'I promise.'

I had to give up my seat on the tube when a Combine got on, dressed head to toe in that unmistakable Combine green, ensuring everyone knew they'd merged. I spent the journey standing beside a woman loudly lamenting to her friend about a man named Jags who still hadn't left his wife.

I tried to tune her out, staring out of the window, and caught the reflection of the Combine who'd taken my seat. The mandala tattoo on their neck was crisp and dark, the ink stark against their skin. I stared until the mandala began to blur, wondering if they'd taken my home as well as my seat.

I thought of Mum, alone in the apartment she despised, growing more unwell and confused with each passing day.

It wasn't until I blinked and felt the wetness on my cheeks that I realised I was crying.

In that moment, I knew I wouldn't be coming back.

I think Albie knew when he was helping me pack.

Albie, unable and unwilling to afford the rent without me, moved back into university accommodation. It was a step back for us, and it meant date nights often became group affairs, with his flatmates noisily tagging along.

One night we went to Hunters, one of the university bars. It was the last philosophy social before UCL broke up for Christmas, and Albie had dragged me along, insisting he couldn't miss it. We stood in line, waiting to be served, as swarms of Combines moved past us to the front of the queue, being served before us and paying half price for their drinks.

Albie was chatting to a guy standing in line with us. They were laughing about one of their professors, Joe someone, and the spitballs that formed in the corners of his mouth whenever he spoke about Plato. I'd met most of the people at the social before but hadn't spoken to many of them. From experience, I knew the boys were on the pull and would lose interest in me as soon as they learned I wasn't single. The girls, whom Albie said were lovely, always seemed bored by me the moment they discovered I worked full-time. 'I get not wanting to study and everything,' they'd say, 'but didn't you want the uni experience?'

When I explained that I'd chosen an apprenticeship so that I could go straight into video production and start earning, their eyes would glaze over. They'd look past me, searching for someone more stimulating to talk to, someone who'd stay out until the early hours and sleep through their 9 a.m. lecture the next day.

Albie insisted the girls liked me, but it was clear they didn't. As we stood in line, none of them spoke to me. When we finally reached the bar, Albie offered to buy my drink. 'What about me, Albs?' Lexi said. None of the girls were particularly friendly, but Lexi made me the most uncomfortable. She had dated Albie when they were at school together and clearly still had a thing for him.

Whoever had organised the social had only booked two tables for sixty people. Most of the society members had to stand. They leaned over one another, shouting above the music. A lanky man with long mousey hair stood behind me. He kept bumping into me and then apologising too loudly in the posh voice he tried hard to suppress. Each time he leaned forward to apologise, I felt his damp breath on my cheek. 'You're fine.' I smiled, rolling up my beer-sodden sleeve.

'Don't worry about it.' When he eventually moved to the other side of the table, he watched me, his eyes lingering for so long that I felt compelled to button my shirt to the neck.

'What about you, Amelia?' Lexi was looking at me, her thumb circling the rim of a beer bottle, the nail painted a chipped, dark burgundy. 'What are you doing about it?'

I watched her thumb, distracted by the uneven polish. I hadn't been involved in her conversation and had no idea what she was talking about. 'Sorry.' I shook my head. 'What am I doing about…?'

'The victims.' Lexi spoke slowly and loudly, as though I were thick, hard of hearing, or both. 'You know, the people being forced into merging against their will…'

'Oh.' I blinked at her, at the faces surrounding her. Five girls, all beautiful, all staring at me expectantly, waiting for my response.

'What am I doing about it?' I let out a nervous laugh. 'I'm… How can I…?'

'Well, we're protesting,' one of the girls said.

'Oh, right. Good for you.' I thought of Mum, her memory slipping away. A wave of futility washed over me.

Lexi tapped her beer bottle against her teeth. 'So, what are you doing to help? I've never seen you at a rally.'

'I do other things,' I said. 'I boycott companies that support Combine. I hand out pamphlets, volunteer at the food bank.' But I could tell from Lexi's expression that it wasn't enough. 'I guess I could protest, too,' I added quickly. 'I was thinking about it, actually.'

The lie hung in the air. The girls exchanged glances, Lexi arching an eyebrow.

My words caught Albie's attention. He turned and took my hand. 'You're coming to the protest?'

'Why not.' I shrugged, aiming for nonchalance.

'Are you sure?' Albie's voice dropped, quiet enough that only I could hear. 'I thought it would be too difficult with your dad and everything.'

'When is it?'

'Saturday.'

I had a wedding to film. It would be impossible for me to make the protest. But it was Lexi's smirk that made me say it. It was Lexi, who never talked to me or looked in my direction unless it was to make me feel small, who inadvertently reintroduced me to the notion of having a voice.

'I'll make it work,' I said. Then I kissed Albie on the mouth just so she'd have to watch. 'I'll be there.'

I left the wedding as soon as the speeches were done. The march was still going on, and Albie had sent me his live location, so I was able to track him. By the time I reached Edgware tube station, he was already in central London. There wasn't time to go back to the flat to change. I arrived at the protest in pressed black trousers, a white shirt and a blazer, my camera bag slung across my chest.

It took longer than I'd anticipated to reach Westminster. So many crazed, furious people meant delays, streets closed off or impassable, police stationed on every corner. I fought my way through the packed Underground station, emerging to more crowds.

The chanting made it easy to locate the march. '*Fuck Combine. Fuck Brightwell. Fuck Combine. Fuck Brightwell.*' There was no let-up, no point at which the crowd tired and lost enthusiasm and the chant became less powerful. I found myself mouthing along before I'd even caught sight of them.

There were flames, explosions, bottles being thrown. Screams and sirens. People barged past me, running towards the centre of the chaos. None of my messages were delivering to Albie, so I relied on the live location to track him down. According to my screen, he was here, right where I stood. I scanned the crowd, but the bodies were so tightly packed that I had no chance of spotting him.

Next to me, a topless man was filming himself, his phone raised high. 'Fuck Combine!' he screamed, panning his phone across the sea of people. I saw then just how far back the crowd stretched, an endless wave of bodies. In the distance, cheers erupted as someone set fire to a makeshift sculpture of Timothy Brightwell, the flames licking at his limbs as the crowd roared in approval.

I pulled out my camera.

Suddenly, I was back there with Dad: my eye pressed to the viewfinder, activists surrounding me. I took photos, hundreds of them, feeling Dad's presence as if he were right beside me, urging me on. My hands shook as I started filming, panning across the crowd, overcome with rage at what had killed him.

Dad had known what the world was coming to. He'd fought to prevent this. And yet, here we were. Without him.

I allowed myself to be swallowed up by the collective fury, chanting until long after my throat was raw.

From that day forward, I started to document everything. I filmed protests, interviewed activists and anti-Mergers. I started shooting Commitment Ceremonies, capturing the Partners on camera before they Committed. 'I like to get to know my clients,' I'd say when they queried the pre-Ceremony interviews. 'It helps to make the film more personal.' I meticulously stored every piece of footage, backing it up on hard drives, organising the clips into folders.

I kept track of the new rules governing the UK. Some, like the mandatory monthly pregnancy tests, were inescapable, relentlessly repeated in advertisements, plastered on the walls of the Underground stations and train carriages. Notifications pinged on our phones on the first of every month – a direct message from the government reminding us to submit our tests before midnight.

Other regulations, like the employment restrictions, were quieter. Slipped into a single announcement and then buried, never mentioned again unless by direct questioning. Government officials remained silent as millions found themselves unable to progress at work, penalised for their non-Combine status or for having large families.

Meanwhile, Combines were quickly promoted, their salaries boosted, as companies rewarded their employees for their sacrifice. Businesses that failed to recognise the superiority of Combines found themselves failing the diversity and inclusion compliance audits.

I joined more anti-Merge groups on social media that kept me up to date with everything the mainstream media was intent on hiding. I reached out to these groups, asking if they'd be willing to speak on camera. Albie and I brainstormed together, deciding what questions to ask and what stories needed to be told.

I saw the ripple effect as families struggled to cope with the financial repercussions of the Merge. I came back from my shifts at the food bank exhausted and frustrated, overwhelmed by the growing demand. 'We didn't have enough supplies to get through even half of the people who needed them. We were turning away desperate kids, telling them there was nothing we could do.' I put my head in my hands. 'These parents, you should have seen them, Mum. They're having to decide between starving their kids or merging them. How do you make that kind of choice?'

There was a period when I thought we were making progress; there was a surge in underground movements advocating for equal employment and healthcare opportunities. Other countries began to take notice. Combine faced mounting international scrutiny, criticised as the world watched the UK grapple with the fallout from its new laws. I hadn't planned what to do with all the footage I'd gathered, and for the first time, I started to hope I wouldn't need to use it. It felt like the world was finally waking up.

Then Combine fought back. They ramped up their propaganda campaign. Timothy Brightwell, Combine's lead investor, became ubiquitous. His silver hair and artificial smile were everywhere, on TV ads, talks shows, podcasts. People who had never chosen to follow him on social media suddenly found themselves subscribed to all his pages.

He relentlessly shared success stories, going on about what the Merge meant for the future of our country. For the future of our world.

Everywhere you went, Combines were treated as elite members of society. They were given priority in every sector, discounts on everyday purchases, significantly reduced mortgage rates. Newspapers were filled with interviews featuring Combines boasting about their newfound privileges. Those of us who remained singular, non-Combines, were demonised. Whenever a crime was committed by a non-Combine, it was emphasised that they were part of the problem due to their inherent selfishness. The effect was such that people who were previously furious about the Merge started to sign up willingly. They wanted to be part of the glorious revolution.

When Mum was offered the Alzheimer's trial, I was outraged. The Merge represented everything I despised. But the more I thought it over, the more I saw my opportunity. By participating in the trial, I could get inside the Clinic. I could document everything, get footage no one has ever had access to. I could find out what really happens within those walls, interview the people desperate enough to put themselves forward for the experiment.

Mum's always valued truth and justice above all else — principles she fought for fiercely in her younger years. In their twenties, she and Mary were regularly involved in protests, lending their voices to causes that mattered. Mum never speaks of it now, and I never witnessed the activist in her myself, but I've seen photographs and I heard the stories from Dad during our own marches.

I often wondered why she stopped, but Dad insisted she hadn't. 'She's still the same,' he'd say, 'she just channels her convictions in quieter ways now, like the way she dedicates herself to her students at the special needs school. She advocates for those kids every single day.'

I knew Mum would never want to merge; the very idea would horrify her. But I couldn't risk telling her the plan, letting her know we were undercover. She had to believe we were truly committed.

All I had to do was get her into the Clinic and through the sessions. Once we completed our preparation, we'd have all the information we needed, and then we'd refuse to proceed. With her unwavering sense of right and wrong, she'd be our way out.

When it was all over — when I revealed the real reason we were there — Mum would be so proud, not just of herself but of us.

But there was one problem. I'd been so vocal in my outrage, so loud within the anti-Merge community, that I needed a solid reason for my sudden change of heart, something convincing enough to make everyone believe I really wanted to go ahead with the experiment.

It needed to be a matter of life or death. Of remembering or forgetting.

Laurie

It's enormously difficult to keep track of these sessions. They blur into one, the circle of metal chairs and white walls forming an endless loop in my mind. It doesn't help that my thoughts are so intent on wandering, drifting back to moments long since past. My notes are hard to make sense of for that reason; so often, I'm not truly in the room. The man's smile is kind, his eyes understanding. He assumes I haven't followed along because of my Alzheimer's, not because my mind is elsewhere. I check his badge. *Nathan, Support Worker.* 'Sorry, Nathan,' I say. 'Could you repeat the question?'

I'm unsure if I was born with a mind intent on escaping or if, as Mary always says, it was a coping mechanism I developed to survive my childhood home. The irony being that my tendency to daydream often landed me in trouble. My mother found it charming, but my stepfather couldn't stand my aloofness. 'She'll never amount to anything,' he'd say. 'Look at her, not a bloody clue. Off in fucking la-la land again.'

'How long ago were you diagnosed?' Nathan asks.

I look around the circle. Amelia isn't here.

'Three years ago,' I tell him. 'But I knew something was wrong long before that. I'd been getting into trouble at work, losing track of things… and I'd get lost, find myself heading somewhere and forgetting why. I knew it was dementia. It was

Amelia who couldn't accept it. She made me retake the tests. The result was the same, of course.'

'Amelia's making you do this, isn't she?' the young girl across from me – Lara, the addict – asks, her voice sharp.

I nod slowly. 'She's intent on saving me. Preserving my memories.'

'And how do you feel about having your memories preserved?' Nathan asks gently.

They all have their eyes on me.

I look down at my notebook, open on my lap. 'I feel sick about it,' I admit. 'I feel sick that Amelia believes she has no choice but to give up her life, her independence, her autonomy, and exist as a Combine to save me—'

'But isn't it beautiful?' a boy's voice interrupts. I look up. *Noah, Participant.* 'Isn't it amazing that Amelia loves you so much? I don't think you should look at it as Amelia losing herself when you merge. That's not how this works. You both get to become a better version of yourself. You become healthy, and she keeps her mother *and* gains all your life experience.' He smiles. 'I was hesitant too when Lucas first told me that he wanted to do this. I felt guilty, thinking he was going to give up his life for me. But here's the thing: he's not. No one's dying. We'll both still be here. I'll still be me, just without the cancer. And you'll still be you, without the dementia.'

Nathan nods approvingly. 'Well said, Noah.'

I look at Noah, at his white cap and matching t-shirt, trying to see the hope he's describing.

'I don't buy it,' Lara says, crossing her arms. 'I don't get how we can still be us when we're sharing someone else's body.'

'It's a tremendously difficult concept to wrap your head around,' Nathan says. 'It's why we have all these months of preparation. The Merge is such a radical procedure, so unlike anything that's been possible before. How can you possibly understand what it's like to merge when you've never experienced anything like it?'

Lara shrugs. 'Noah gets it.'

'And you will, too, Lara. Just give it time. How are you feeling today? Any more optimistic?'

Lara mumbles something under her breath, her words so soft and slurred that I have trouble understanding her. After a few minutes of failed listening, I give up and start jotting down some quick notes before the thoughts escape me.

> *No one disappearing. Amelia still here. Me still here.*
> *No dementia!*
> *How can we still be us when we're sharing someone else's body?*

I refocus on Lara, straining to make sense of her rushed words. 'Dad's been sitting with me when I've been doing my grounding exercises,' she says, her eyes fixed on her scuffed, worn-out trainers, the laces frayed. 'He sits there, watching me, making sure I'm doing it properly. How can I exist in the same body as someone who has so little faith in me?'

She shifts in her chair, pulling one leg up under herself, and that's when I see them – marks, faint burns, scarring the top of her inner thigh.

I'm helping Amelia at work today. Properly helping her. It's not like the times I've come to film with a malfunctioning brain, when I've stood behind the camera, convinced I'm capturing everything, only to discover later that I stopped filming a few minutes in or forgot to press Record altogether. Today, I feel like my old self.

The village hall has been transformed. It no longer resembles a place where council meetings are held, Girl Guides gather, or mums and toddlers meet. A large wrought-iron arch, decorated with foliage and white roses, stands at the main entrance. From the arch, an ankle-deep river of white petals flows down the centre of the hall, widening into a large pool at the far end. Wooden stools are arranged in three concentric circles within the pool of petals, each topped with a round white linen cushion. In the centre, a small wooden platform holds two dark-green cushions, each embroidered with the Combine mandala.

'I wonder how much this all cost,' I say, my eyes wandering to the ceiling beams, wrapped in fairy lights, white roses, purple hyssop and green laurel leaves. 'Mary's goddaughter got married last year. Little Rachel. Do you remember her? With the lovely ginger hair. Her wedding cost tens of thousands. For a small service, too. Nothing fancy.'

'This isn't a wedding, Mum.' Amelia's been short with me all morning. I tried broaching the subject of alternative treatments, but she refuses to hear it. She's adamant that we see this through. I called her belligerent, and she's only proving my point.

'I understand that, Amelia. I'm just saying, Rachel's wedding was far less lavish than this Ceremony appears to be, and it still cost an arm and a leg.'

She stops fiddling with her camera and finally looks at me. 'You don't have to pay anything so long as you agree to use the traditional trappings.'

'All this is free?'

She nods. 'Combine pays for it because it makes the whole ordeal feel more like a celebration. The more people who see it being celebrated like this, all luxurious and exciting, the more people will want to merge. Read through your notes before the Ceremony starts, Mum. All the information is in there.'

As Amelia heads off to film some location shots, I get my notebook from my bag. It's the specific one I always bring to Ceremonies, containing all the information I need: details on how the cameras work, the sequence of events during the service and the expected behaviour once it begins. Even on days like today, when I feel like I've remembered everything, I check. It's so easy to forget the rules, to miss something important.

I flip open the notebook and scan the list on the first page.

1. *Check camera settings and battery level*

2. *Set up in a discreet location to capture Ceremony*

3. *Pay attention to the positioning of Witnesses (friends and family). Inner circle = more shots needed*

4. *Capture candid moments and reactions from the attendees, especially during key emotional points in the Ceremony*

5. *Sequence of events:*
   - *Witnesses stand, Circle of Support is opened*
   - *Partners under arch – walk down aisle into Circle of Support*
   - *Promise of the Witnesses (bow head for this part)*
   - *Thanksgiving*
   - *Blessings and wishes*
   - *Conclusion and celebration*
   - *Partners leave for Merge*
   - *Reception and festivities*

At the bottom of the page is a note written in Amelia's handwriting: *Not everyone chooses to Commit. Don't assume they are doing this by choice.*

I study the room, trying to gauge whether these Partners have truly chosen to Commit or if they've been coerced. The guests, congregating in the middle of the hall, seem happy enough. They chat excitedly in small groups on either side of the aisle of petals.

Amelia moves along the perimeter of the hall, her knees bent slightly, the camera outstretched in front of her as she captures every detail. She's focused on the framed stencil art lining the walls. I look at the frame closest to me: a couple walking hand in hand down a tree-lined path, fallen leaves lining their way. I reach out, letting my finger trace the glass, following the etched cursive spiralling up the trunk of a tree: *The Ultimate Commitment.*

The next frame contains a stencil of the same couple standing on a beach, gazing up at the night sky. *All of me, all of you, all of us* curls its way around the full moon.

Somehow, even on the days when I've messed up, forgotten to record, missed crucial moments, Amelia manages to create something beautiful. She's clever with the moments she chooses to include. The Partners are always smiling, never showing stress or doubt. The Witnesses are full of energy, laughing and dancing, never worried or hesitant. Amelia's films make the day look so much like a fairy tale that I often cry when watching the finished productions.

A hush falls over the room as a Combine dressed in a floor-length, forest-green robe steps through the archway. The Officiant. They smile as they move down the aisle of petals. 'Good afternoon,' they say, their voice amplified through the small microphone clipped to their robe. 'Please take your seats.'

Noise fills the room again as the Witnesses move towards their stools. I return to my camera, feeling the familiar bubbles of excitement popping in my stomach. As the Witnesses settle, the Officiant approaches those seated directly in line with the aisle. 'I need the six of you to open the circle,' they instruct, showing two guests on each ring where to reposition their stools. 'This is only for the entrance, of course. Once Helena and Samuel are in the centre, I'll need you to move the stools back to their original positions and secure the Circle of Support before the Promise of the Witnesses begins.'

The chosen Witnesses smile proudly, thrilled to have been given the task of closing the circle. I wonder if it's their first Ceremony and they unknowingly chose the stools in line with the aisle, or if they deliberately selected their seats, eager to secure the circle round their loved ones.

Amelia has asked me to film the Partners as they enter the hall. She'll be capturing it too, but from a different angle. I'm responsible for the close-ups, a task I gladly accepted. Watching the Partners beneath the arch is my favourite part of the Ceremony. There's something so intimate about seeing their reactions as they lift their eyes and take in the Circle of Support waiting for them at the end of the aisle. Sometimes they break down in tears. Sometimes they lift their veils and kiss. Sometimes they just stand there, mutely taking it all in.

I position my camera to practise my second shot. Once the Partners move on from the archway, I'm to focus on the centre of the circle, on the two dark-green cushions where the Partners will kneel. My job is to film their growing anticipation, capturing any shared glances, any silent communication.

I pan slowly along the outer circle. Most of the women wear simple white dresses, while the men are in plain white suits, complete with white ties and gloves. The younger girls have white ribbons in their hair, cascading in curls from their ponytails. The boys wear white shirts and shorts, white socks and white shoes. I continue to move the camera until I reach the first guest wearing green. A Combine. I linger on them as they talk to the man next to them. Other than their green clothes, there's nothing to suggest they're any different from everyone else. Perhaps they aren't.

I shift the camera to focus on the Officiant, standing on the little platform behind the cushions. They have a male appearance and are probably in their thirties. I wonder if this is their actual age, or just how they appear now. What were they like before? Have they always looked like a man? Is the beard a new addition or something they've kept? I zoom in on their eyes until they take up the majority of the frame. Brown, narrow, slightly bloodshot. They're squinting, looking past the camera. 'Where are you?' I whisper. 'Are you in there? Can you see me?'

The Officiant's eyes narrow further, almost vanishing entirely as the soft, lilting music begins to play. The Witnesses rise from their stools, linking arms across shoulders to form three concentric arcs; the curved, white chains resemble a rainbow, open and inviting. I zoom out, moving the camera back to its original position in front of the arch, adjusting the focus before hitting Record.

The Partners appear, hand in hand, their heads bowed beneath their veils. They pause beneath the arch. They're dressed in ceremonial robes identical to the Officiant's, except theirs are a deep, rich purple. In their free hands, they each hold a bouquet of white roses.

The Officiant raises their arms. 'Honoured are you, Our Combines, who sacrifice your future for the future of our world.'

'We honour those who sacrifice themselves for the survival of tomorrow,' the Witnesses respond, their arms still draped around one another's shoulders.

The Partners, standing beneath the arch, raise their heads and lift each other's veils. The man lets out a sound – a soft, trembling whimper – not quite a cry, but something close. The woman remains silent, her expression steady. Together, they look down the aisle at their Circle of Support, which looks back at them. The gentle music fades and is replaced by the brass- and percussion-heavy strains of the Commitment March.

The Partners walk slowly down the aisle, their long purple robes sweeping petals aside. Some cling stubbornly to the fabric, carried along with them. As they near the circle, the Witnesses bow their heads in respect.

Behind my camera, I do the same.

Amelia

Albie's here. He's in the kitchen, his low tones interspersed with Mum's high-pitched laughter. He's always known how to make her laugh. The first time they met, his impersonation of Our Combine had her in tears at the dinner table. He wobbled his head as he spoke, the way they do. The way we presumed all Combines would.

'It – is – my – greatest – honour – to – force – you – into – this – hideous – existence – and – speak – like – a – mal – func – tion – ing – ro – bot.'

Mum wiped her eyes and snorted. 'You're cruel,' she said, still laughing. 'But you're pitch-perfect. They do sound bizarre, don't they? I've not liked to mention how odd they are, considering what they're doing for our planet, but why *does* their head move like that? As though their neck is a spring. Do it again, Albie. Go on. It's so funny.'

Albie smiled and squeezed my knee beneath the table, a silent celebration of securing Mum's approval. Mum's affection for him has only grown in the years since. She was the one who invited him over today, insisting he join her for a walk. She appeared at my bedroom door, leaning against the frame with her phone pressed to her ear, her cardigan draped loosely over her shoulders. I quickly closed the video I was editing and opened some footage from a wedding I filmed last year.

'Amelia's busy editing,' Mum said into the phone, 'and I fancy getting some fresh air. Walk with me, won't you, Albie? I'll treat you to an ice cream.'

She laughed loudly, her cardigan slipping from one shoulder, and my stomach twisted with a longing to be part of their joke, to join them on the walk, to talk to Albie properly – tell him about the sessions, the Support Workers, about Lara, who desperately doesn't want to be there. I want to confide in him like I used to, to ask for his advice, to show him the edit I've started putting together. With each passing week, the need to unburden myself to Albie grows. But I can't. To involve him would be to pull him into something that isn't his, something that could compromise his safety.

Albie's already been arrested twice. Both times he was defending the rights of non-Combines, and both times they let him go with only a stern warning. But the authorities were clear: a third arrest would mean serious consequences. *Prison overcrowding necessitates merging of inmates,* the announcement said. *We trust in your support as we address the challenges posed by our growing population.* Another arrest could have Albie sentenced. Merged against his will.

Mum hung up and told me Albie was coming over. I texted to thank him. He knows how easily Mum loses her bearings these days, how she now prefers having company when she walks. He was probably busy, but he would have insisted he was free and that he fancied nothing more than getting ice cream with her.

I join them in the kitchen. Albie's leaning on the counter, his lips pressed tightly together. 'The remarkable thing is,' Mum's saying, 'Amelia never said those words in that order. We had to record certain sounds, and some words and phrases, and then they stitched them together using phonetics. I know I have my scepticisms regarding all this "merging", but I must say, this part is thoroughly enjoyable. The wonders of modern technology.'

Mum's earpieces are just about visible in Albie's ears. He taps his finger against one of them, adjusting the volume. 'God. It's so realistic.'

Mum scans the open notebook in her lap. 'It says here that I should now be wearing them for two hours twice a day. Then the time I'm required to wear them increases until, eventually, I'm wearing them all day.'

Albie removes the earpieces and places them on the counter. 'Thank you for showing me, Lor. That's really—' He notices me. 'Hi,' he says.

'Hi.' I approach him slowly and kiss him gently on the cheek. He doesn't move, his body tense. Mum's busy putting the earpieces in, too focused on the task to notice the stiffness between us.

'Your mum's been filling me in on your latest sessions.'

Mum nods. 'You haven't told Albie much about the Clinic, Amelia. The poor boy had no idea what we've been up to. I've been reading through my notes. We've done such a lot in such a short amount of time. It's no wonder I'm exhausted.'

I open a cupboard and begin rummaging for a snack I don't need. 'You're not meant to talk about the sessions, Mum.'

She rolls her eyes. 'Nothing's confidential among family. It's like with Mary. She's not meant to tell me anything about the patients at the hospital, but she does. Of course she does. Just last week a man mistook a bottle of nail polish remover for eyedrops. Mary said his eyes looked like two ripe tomatoes.' She laughs loudly. 'You couldn't write it.'

I rip open a packet of crisps.

'Your mum mentioned there's a speaker coming soon. You'll get the chance to talk to them, to find out what it's really like being a Combine.'

I nod, munching slowly. 'Rosa-Liam. They're Callie's brother.'

'Callie?'

'She's one of the Support Workers.'

Mum flaps her hand at us. 'Could you two be quiet? It's so difficult to concentrate on the recording when you're speaking.'

'That's the point, Mum. You're supposed to get used to hearing my voice along with everyone else's.'

She's frowning at me. 'I didn't know you'd been to Portugal. Who did you go with? Isn't there lots of trouble going on there at the moment? All that rioting?'

'I haven't been to Portugal, Mum.'

'Then why are you talking about your visit to the Belem Tower in Lisbon?'

Albie's watching me again, his gaze steady and probing. I fiddle with the crisp packet, pretending to read the label. Without a word, he takes me by the arm and leads me through to the next room.

'This isn't good for her,' he says, his voice low. 'This whole thing is only going to worsen her confusion. Surely you can see that, Amelia.'

I crush the crisp packet in my hand, unable to meet his eyes. Seeing Mum so confused, so lost in the recordings, overwhelmed by the constant flood of information from the sessions, is hard enough without Albie bringing it up.

'I know you don't want your mum to get worse, but putting her through all of this for an experiment that might not even work...'

I glance up at him, but it's too difficult. What am I supposed to say? What I want is to scream that of course I don't want her to get worse, that the very thought of her slipping away terrifies me. But the reality is, she *will* get worse. I know that.

No matter what I do, her decline is inevitable. What I want, what I'm trying so hard to do, is to give her the chance to be part of something bigger, something meaningful – something that might just outlast her memories.

The silence stretches. Then: 'Why are you doing this, Mills?'

'I can't go through this again. You know why I'm doing it.'

'But it's so fucking short-sighted.' He grips my shoulders. 'You were a fucking anti-Merger, Amelia. For years. What was all of that for?'

'Things were different then.' I finally meet his eyes. 'Keep your voice down, Albie. Please.'

'You're going to be taking on her confusion,' he says, quieter, but no less intense, 'muddling up your own mind for the tiniest chance she'll clear hers. And you'll be supporting these greedy bastards by doing it. Going against everything you believe in.'

I shake my head. 'It's not all bad, Albie. You should see how Lucas talks about saving Noah, or how desperate Annie and Ben are to start their family, or how terrified Jay is of losing Lara. It's not as black and white as we once thought. There are situations that justify the Merge. I know it's flawed and messed up. But, Albs, it does some good too.'

He shakes his head, his hands now covering his mouth as if my words might make him sick. The nausea twists inside me, too. I can't believe what I've just said. The words came so easily. Too easily. I scramble for something else, some excuse to make me feel less conflicted.

'It's what Dad would have wanted,' I blurt.

Albie lowers his hands. 'What?'

My throat tightens, my eyes sting. It's been ten years, but Dad's death hasn't got any easier to talk about. I feel terrible now for using his memory this way.

'I should have been with him that day,' I say, my voice trembling. 'I should've gone, and I didn't. I could have saved him. He wouldn't have put himself in danger if I'd been there. He'd have been careful. He'd have looked after me... he'd still be alive.'

'Amelia...'

'When I merge with Mum, I'll be doing my bit to repair the world, and I'll be saving her too. I'll be protecting the two things Dad cared about most. I've got to make it up to him, Albie. I have to show him how sorry I am for leaving him alone that day.'

But the truth is, Dad would never have wanted this. He'd have been outside the Clinic, holding a placard alongside the protestors. He'd have marched until his legs gave out, standing firm against everything I'm now defending. Shame presses down on my chest until I can hardly breathe.

Albie lowers his gaze, his jaw tightening. 'It's not your fault your dad died,' he says. 'You can't carry that with you forever.'

'Go on the walk with Mum,' I say quietly. 'I love you, Albs. And I'm sorry.' I kiss his cheek. 'Thank you so much for walking with her.'

The Merge was first suggested to us during Mum's annual check-up. We'd scarcely been in the doctor's office a few minutes when I realised things were worse than we'd hoped. The tests Mum had taken in the weeks prior showed significant progression of her Alzheimer's. Her scores in memory and recognition tests had plummeted. They would alter her medication and see if that helped slow the progression, but beyond that there was nothing more they could do.

'Except,' the doctor said, her voice calm, her white coat perfectly crisp, the sleeves neatly folded. 'Have you ever considered the Merge?'

I blinked, my eyes hot. 'What?'

'The Merge,' she repeated, just as calmly.

Mum's face reddened. 'How dare you,' she said. 'How dare you suggest such a thing. Aren't you supposed to be consoling me, offering support and advice? You've just delivered the worst news there could be and followed it up with a suggestion that I...' She looked at me, her voice faltering, tears spilling down her cheeks.

I stood up, taking Mum's hand. 'Come on, Mum. We don't need to stay and listen to this.'

We'd been so positive in the run-up to that appointment, repeatedly reassuring each other that her dementia wasn't anywhere near as bad as everyone said it would be. But after the news, Mum struggled to keep it together.

Albie was staying over the night she had her biggest meltdown. We'd gone to bed. Mum was in the bathroom with the shower on and the taps running, trying her best to cover the sound of her sobs, but they were so loud they woke us up.

Albie sat up, rubbing his eyes. He listened for a moment, then jumped out of bed and pulled on his jeans. 'She sounds like she needs help, Amelia.'

'Don't,' I whispered, reaching for his arm. 'Please, Albie, she can't know that we can hear her.'

I pressed my fists into my eyes. Albie hesitated, then climbed back into bed and pulled me in to him. He stroked my hair, and the kindness of it made it impossible to stop my tears.

I imagined Mum in the bathroom, holding a towel to her face. She'd never had a meltdown with a visitor in the apartment before. It had always been just me, and I'd done a good job of pretending I hadn't heard a thing – like the night she spent hours pacing the hallway, crying. The next morning, she was in the kitchen making breakfast, her face perfectly composed as if nothing had happened. We sat together, talking about the day ahead as though the night hadn't left her in pieces.

I pulled away from Albie and wiped my eyes. 'If she knows that I can hear her, then she'll only get more upset. She never lets herself be sad around me, not even when Dad died. The only time I ever see her vulnerable is when she forgets. All the time she's lucid, which is most of the time, she only ever shows frustration. Never sadness. Never fear.'

'That's sad, Amelia.'

I gestured at the door. 'It's fucking devastating, Albie.'

I got back under the covers. Albie stayed where he was, his jeans half-pulled up, perching next to me. He stroked my back as I cried into the pillow. The shower stopped. I looked up at Albie. Both of us went quiet, trying to follow Mum's slow footsteps down the hall. I waited for the sound of her bedroom door closing.

'Amelia?' Her voice came from outside my door. 'Amelia?'

Albie stood and quickly buttoned his jeans. I wiped my eyes and flattened my hair. 'Come in, Mum,' I said.

She hovered in the doorway, reluctant to enter. Her mauve nightie was inside out and back to front, the label jutting out beneath her chin. 'Oh, Mum.' I got out of bed, pulling down my t-shirt, and hurried to her. I took her in my arms, and she rested her forehead on my shoulder. Albie mouthed that he'd be in the lounge. He squeezed past us and slipped out of the room.

I held Mum close.

'I don't know what's wrong with me. I don't know why my brain isn't working. I'm... I'm...' But no words came, just tears.

I led her over to the bed, and she sat cross-legged on the duvet. I took her hand.

'What am I going to do? I don't want to forget. I don't want to forget you. I can't forget you.'

'You won't forget me, Mum.'

'I will,' she said simply. 'I have dementia. I will forget you, Amelia.'

She looked nothing like herself in that moment, slouched and pale, her hair a messy tangle. 'I don't want it to get worse, but I don't know how to stop it. My head… it feels… it's like it doesn't belong to me anymore.'

'Mum, you have to trust that the new medication will help. That's what it does, it prevents the disease from progressing. It stops it from getting worse.'

'But for how long?'

She looked so tired, so worn down. I pulled back the duvet, and she crawled into bed like a child. It didn't take long for her to fall asleep. She looked so small beneath the covers, so unlike herself. I draped my arm over her, and she nestled closer.

I will forget you, Amelia.

I knew that she was right. She would forget me. But perhaps I could make sure that, even long after she was gone, the world would never forget her.

Amelia

We go over to Annie and Ben's on Friday night. Their apartment is larger than ours, and it's clear they've taken the time to decorate. The walls are freshly painted, the furniture matching. I come prepared to help serve food and fill glasses, but Annie won't allow me to return the favour. 'Ben's a perfectionist,' she says when I offer to help with the cooking. 'We're all better off leaving him to it. Lara and Noah are being brave and keeping him company.'

Annie raises her eyebrows and looks towards the kitchen, where Ben's voice rings out over a clattering of pots and pans. 'Show tunes, no less. When I popped in earlier, he was using a wooden spoon as a microphone and belting out some ballad from *Phantom of the Opera*. I don't think that's something you want to get involved in.' She nods at the camera I've brought along. 'Are you our photographer for the night?'

'I came straight from an engagement shoot. Thought I'd bring it in and take some photos. Or videos. In fact, I might just have to capture Ben's performance.'

I get footage of everyone chatting and laughing, of Lara sulking. Of her first smile, brought on by the sight of Mum. Ellie and Kath are here too. Lucas is so eager to introduce Ellie that he stumbles over his words. 'Ellie, this is Amelia and Mum – Lor... told you about.'

Ellie laughs and hugs us both. 'It's so lovely to meet you,' she says.

'Likewise.' I smile. 'I've heard so much about you.'

Kath is more reserved, her eyes rarely leaving Lara, as if she's afraid to let her daughter out of sight for even a moment. 'I'm so excited for you all,' Ellie keeps saying. 'All Combines are amazing, obviously, but you lot are the game-changers. I couldn't believe it when Lucas and Noah were selected. You've all done so well to be chosen.'

My phone chimes with Mum's medication reminder, and I put my camera away. We sneak off to the nursery so that she can take her pills in private. She stares at the wall as I prepare the medication, running her finger along the pink and orange swirls with a distant look.

'Annie painted the room herself,' I tell her. 'Isn't it beautiful?'

'People usually go with yellow or beige when they don't know the baby's gender,' she says, still studying the paintwork. 'This is very refreshing, Amelia. It's fun. It shows exactly what kind of parents they'll be.' She looks around, taking in the antique-style baby crib in the corner, the cloud-shaped rug in the middle of the floor and the toybox by the door, already filled, the lid propped open to show the teddies. I have no doubt that, if I opened the drawers, they'd be neatly filled with folded babygrows and nappies. 'It really is lovely in here,' Mum says.

I pass her the pills. 'Remember to eat something when we go back into the other room. The tablets don't do well on an empty stomach.'

Mum smirks as she tips the pills into her mouth.

'What?' I say, passing her a glass of water.

She swallows. 'You sound like a right old nag.'

'I'm just looking after you, Mum.'

'I know, and I love you for it. But you must admit it's funny. You hated me nagging you and now here you are, going on at me to eat.' Mum hands me back the empty pill container, and I put it in my bag. It's a handbag, but it feels more like a knapsack. I'm like a new mum who can't leave the house without a mountain of spare clothes and snacks.

Mum places her palm on an orange swirl. 'How long do we have left?'

'Until we merge?'

She nods.

'Six weeks.'

She drops her hand and wanders over to the crib. 'I'm really not sure about all of this, Amelia. What these people are doing, I'm not sure I agree with it.'

'Which people?'

She frowns, fingering the white lace border of the crib. 'What if the baby doesn't make it?'

'Don't say that. Of course the baby will make it.'

'But what if it doesn't?' She grips the railings of the crib. 'What happens then? You shouldn't build a nursery before the baby arrives, Amelia. It makes everything unbearably difficult afterwards. Even if you're lucky enough to have a healthy baby, there's no guarantee they'll stay that way. You can do everything in your power to keep them safe, and still... they can get sick. Isn't it terrible?'

She lets go of the railings and cradles her own stomach, as though she's the one expecting a child. I pull her hands gently away. 'Don't do that, Mum,' I say. 'Let's go back to the lounge, shall we?'

Mum's been cradling her stomach every time she reads her notes about Annie and Ben. We went food shopping at the weekend, and she wandered around, her hand on her tummy, smiling at the secret of her pregnancy.

'There's something wrong,' she says, her eyes wide with panic.

I rest my hand gently on her back. I wish there were a guidebook for this, a clear set of instructions: *How to break it to your not-pregnant mother that her baby is okay.* Is this one of those instances in which it's better to break their spell and bring them back to reality?

'You're okay, Mum.'

She turns quickly. Her expression is fearful, as though she doesn't recognise me. 'It's my fault,' she says. 'I should have been more careful with him.'

I shake my head, my throat constricting. 'None of this is your fault.'

'The people in the circle don't get angry. Even when I refuse to get out from under the chair.'

'That's good, Mum.'

'The woman with the missing teeth has them in a ziplock bag. She carries them with her because she can't afford to get them fixed.' She looks at me, her eyes shining. 'It's so sad, isn't it, what people go through?'

She lets her tears spill, something she'd never have allowed before she was unwell. I wipe her cheeks, catching the tears, an ache settling in my chest. What is she thinking about? What has she read or watched that she believes to be real? I hear Eliza's voice, what she's been telling me for over a month now. *You will ensure she never experiences this level of confusion again, Amelia.*

Not for the first time, I find myself wondering: What if we really did this? What if we went through with it and I prevented the inevitable sadness that will consume Mum's life if we remain separate?

I push the thought away.

'It's dreadful, Mum,' I say.

*

We remain in the nursery until Mum seems to have recovered. It doesn't take too long. I distract her by directing her attention back to the walls. 'I like how colourful it is,' she says, her finger following the pink and orange swirls again. 'Most people opt for neutral colours these days. This is far more fun.'

When we return to the lounge, we find everyone laughing together. 'Did Ben's singing drive you out of the kitchen, Noah?' Annie says. 'I apologise in advance if I become a big fan of musicals after the Merge. Please just know that it's Ben, not me. I've far better taste.'

'Oh shit.' Noah groans. 'I hadn't considered music. I'll be playing the fucking trombone in big band.'

Lucas shoves him. 'Just because you couldn't get past Grade Two on the clarinet.'

Ellie giggles. 'You played clarinet? After all the crap you've given us, it turns out you're just a bitter, rejected big-band member. Don't worry, Noah. You can live out your orchestral dreams soon enough.'

Mum wanders off to the dining room. I excuse myself and follow her. She's at the table, filling a small bowl with mixed nuts. I smile. She's remembered to eat.

'Are you okay, Mum?'

She looks at me with wide, startled eyes. 'Mum?' She hesitates for a second, then lowers her voice. 'You know about the baby? You won't say anything, will you, Mary?'

Mary?

The name takes the air from my lungs. Mum has never mistaken me for Mary before. Through it all – through the fog, the forgetting, the repeating – she's always known who I am. I've always been Amelia. I've always been her daughter.

I will away my tears, blinking hard.

'Don't get upset,' she says, her voice soft and conspiratorial, as though we're sharing some secret. 'It's just, I'd hate for Mitch to get his hopes up again.'

Again?

I shake my head, my throat thick. 'I won't say a word.'

Lara sulks into the room and slumps onto one of the chairs, burying her head in her hands. 'They're insufferable,' she groans. 'Mum's in there talking about the fact she got the M.O. like it was some fucking heroic act. It wasn't like they wanted any more kids. She didn't need her womb any more. There was nothing heroic about them removing it. She did it for the money, like we haven't already got enough. You know we've not had to leave our house, right? We're still able to afford our home.'

'What's the M.O.?' Mum asks.

'The Moral Operation,' Lara says. 'Don't worry about remembering it, Lor. There's nothing moral about it. They take your womb and pay you for it.' She looks from Mum to me and back again. 'You're so lucky to have each other, do you know that? You're friends as well as family, aren't you? I can tell.'

'We're best friends.' Mum smiles.

I nod.

'My mum doesn't even like me.'

'I'm sure that's not true. I'm sure your mother loves you very much.'

'Maybe. But she doesn't like me.' Lara stands and moves to the table. She fills a small bowl with crisps and carries it back to her chair. 'She acts like she would have done this with me if we were compatible. She acts like she'd willingly merge with me. There's no fucking way she would. It was the luckiest day of her life when our results came back and we weren't a match.' She shoves a handful of crisps into her mouth. 'She spends all this time watching me now, checking I'm wearing my earpieces, making sure I'm eating healthily and getting to bed at a good time so that I have energy for the sessions. She's never paid any attention to me before. Not really. You know how I hid drugs from them for all those years? I stuffed them in the soft toys she bought me every birthday and Christmas. Fucking soft toys. Who buys soft toys for anyone over the age of ten? And then doesn't find it weird that they're arranged in families all over their seventeen-year-old daughter's room?' She shakes her head. 'They never even found them. They think they saved me, but they had nothing to do with it. I got rid of the drugs myself. I made the choice to get clean.'

Jay laughs loudly in the other room, and Lara closes her eyes.

Mum sits down beside her, and Lara rests her head on Mum's shoulder. 'You're so strong,' Mum says, stroking Lara's hair the way she always does mine. 'You made the decision to get sober and you've stuck to it. If other people want to claim they're the reason for your success, then let them. You know the truth, and that's what matters. We know it too, don't we, Mary?'

My stomach sinks.

'Yes,' I say. 'We believe in you, Lara.'

Lara lifts her head from Mum's shoulder, her eyes welling with fresh tears. 'Thank you,' she whispers. 'I believe in you guys, too.'

In that moment, I see the shift in her, the softening of the disdain she's carried all these weeks. I think she finally understands why we've chosen to be part of this experiment she despises, why I would do anything, risk anything, to keep Mum with me for as long as I can. And, for the first time, I understand it too. I see what the others in this group have seen all along: the fierce, fragile hope that makes this choice feel less like desperation and more like love.

But as I watch Mum now, I can't help but wonder: what if this – her calling me Mary – is the beginning of the end? What if, from this point on, the moments of clarity grow rarer, the forgetting more frequent? What if, one day, she doesn't just forget my name but forgets the essence of me? The laughter we've shared. The love that binds us.

Now that it feels real, I'm not sure I could survive it.

Maybe I don't have to.

Laurie

The sad girl has become quite attached to me. She's started sitting next to me in the circle and at lunch, waiting around to walk with me past the protestors when it's time to go home; she likes to link her arm in mine and hurry me past them, shielding me from their shouts.

When Amelia and the other Hosts left the room just now, the girl shifted her chair closer to mine and I got a whiff of her vanilla perfume. I raised my hand to ask where Amelia was going, and she hushed the room for me. 'Lor has a question,' she said. I can't recall the answer as to where the others have gone, only the girl's unexpected kindness.

The girl is walking beside me now, holding my arm as we follow a woman in a purple tunic down a long corridor. We pass the old hotel rooms. I wonder what's left of them, if they still contain a bed and an ensuite, or if they've been converted into something more practical. Offices, perhaps, for the workers. There are many of them, all dressed in purple.

Mitchell and I always meant to stay here for an anniversary or a birthday, but we never managed it. Something important always got in the way of our plans, the way important things tend to. He'd be so proud of me for being here now, for getting Amelia inside. I must remember to treat her to room service. That was always the plan: tea and pancakes in bed before spending the day wandering around town, playing tourist.

'You must never put off anything,' I tell the girl. 'You must find reasons to go through with your plans as opposed to finding reasons not to.' I check her name badge. 'Is there anything you've always wanted to do, Lara?'

She shrugs. 'I don't know what I want. No one else trusts me to think for myself, so why should I?'

The woman in the purple tunic stops walking, and we halt behind her. She looks at us the way I used to look at my pupils before we entered the hall for an assembly, ensuring everyone was silent and attentive. 'This first visit is just for you to understand the room and to get accustomed to the mirrors,' she says. 'Next week, we'll turn on the projections and begin the acclimatisation process.'

I frown at Lara, wondering about her apparent lack of self-worth. She takes the look to mean I'm not understanding what the woman's talking about. She's right, of course. But that concerns me far less than a young girl not trusting her own mind.

'We're getting used to what we'll look like as a Combine,' she says quietly. 'We'll stick together in there, Lor. Don't worry.'

The room reminds me of the hall of mirrors that Amelia used to love at the fair. She'd drag us in, and we'd walk around laughing at our distorted reflection. Neither Mitchell nor I enjoyed rides, so we were happy to spend our time making silly faces in the mirrors and listening to Amelia's delicious giggles. I look around for her, but she doesn't seem to be here.

'The Room of Reflection,' the woman says proudly, 'is a new incentive set up by Combine following the feedback we received from Participants who reported severe distress when coming to terms with their new bodies. In here, you'll spend time getting used to your new reflection so that life post-Merge is less daunting, less of an adjustment. For each of you here, this shouldn't be too harrowing an experience as you already know and love your Hosts. You're already incredibly familiar with their bodies.'

Lara grunts.

'Spend time walking around the room. As you can see, the mirrors aren't anything to be nervous about. It's only your reflection looking back at you for now. It's a good idea to familiarise yourself with the room, so if you do become anxious later on you can remind yourself how it felt beforehand. Remember, for the next six weeks, the projections aren't reality.'

As we move about the room, no one makes funny faces or laughs. I watch as the poorly boy strokes the frame of a large circular mirror. 'So,' he says, 'next week, when the projections are on, I'll look in here and see Lucas?'

'Yes,' the woman says. 'Depending on which mirror you look in, you'll see a different projection mirroring your actions. Each mirror will provide you with a different experience of your new image. In one, you may be confronted with your new image smartly dressed and put together. In another, you may be in your pyjamas or a football kit covered in mud. The projections are designed to provide you with a unique and accurate reflection of your new image.'

'Epic.' The boy moves quickly to the next mirror, grinning with excitement.

'In some,' the woman continues, 'you will see your Host's naked body reflected. This can be challenging at first, but becoming familiar with your future body in its purest form is essential if you wish to ease your anxieties post-Merge.'

Beside me, Lara stares blankly at her reflection, waiting for it to distort. The mirror we're looking into, with its thick silver frame, reaches almost to the ceiling.

'I don't think it's one of those funny mirror places,' I say gently. 'I think it's just regular reflections. Perhaps we're supposed to admire the frames.' Lara doesn't respond. I try to distract her by pointing out the different shapes and sizes of the mirrors, but she remains fixated on her own image, searching for something in the reflection, something she can't seem to find.

'I don't know how I'm going to do this, Lor,' she says after a while. 'I don't want to look in these mirrors and see him. Why Eliza still thinks I love him is beyond me. I've told her so many times that I hate his fucking guts. I didn't before all of this. But now I do. I really fucking hate him.'

We move to another mirror and stand side by side, our reflections multiplying before us. There are so many versions of ourselves. I scratch my head, and all my reflections mimic me. 'I know it's hard,' I say. 'But maybe this is a chance for you to confront your feelings. To really see yourself. Perhaps that's the purpose of this room. It's not often that we have the opportunity to observe ourselves from every angle. Maybe this room will help you better understand your mind.'

She snorts. 'How is seeing my hideous reflection going to help me understand myself?'

'Hideous? You're not hideous, Lara. Quite the opposite.' I squeeze her hand, and my reflections do the same. 'Just take it one day at a time. We're all in this together, and who knows? If you spend enough time in here, maybe one day you'll look in these mirrors and be happy with what you see.'

She smiles weakly. 'You've forgotten, haven't you?'

I frown at her, the real her, not the one in the mirror. 'Forgotten what?'

'Where we are. What we're doing. I'm merging with my dad, Lor. It'll be him I see in the mirrors.'

My frown deepens, confusion rising like fog. 'Your father? But... what do you mean? Whyever would he be in the mirror?'

Her eyes hold mine. 'How did your mum get through it?' she asks. 'What did she do to get over her addiction?'

I blink. I hadn't realised this girl knew about my mother's drinking. I hadn't realised anyone knew, except Mary.

'Sorry,' she says. 'That's personal. I shouldn't have asked.'

'She never managed to,' I say quietly. 'She had a difficult life, and the alcohol made everything easier for her. It numbed her pain. So, she kept drinking.' I think of my mother, bruised and swollen, fresh blood surfacing on her cut lip as she stretched her mouth into a smile. 'Mummy's okay, Lor,' she'd say, lifting the bottle of vodka. 'This special drink makes all Mummy's pain go away.'

'Do you think I could do it?' Lara asks.

I stare at her, the fog swirling back in.

She looks in the mirror again. 'My dad thinks he's saving me by doing this. He thinks he'll make me stop. I haven't touched the stuff in months, but he's still convinced I'm addicted. Maybe I am. Maybe I always will be.'

'Your dad brought you here, to this room, to scare you out of your addiction?'

She nods. 'He thinks this is the only way to help me.'

'I don't think scaring someone works,' I say. 'At least, it didn't work for my mother. She was always scared. I think that was a big part of her problem.'

I think of him – his smile, his rough hands that held me too tightly.

We stand in front of the mirror for a few more minutes, both lost in thought. 'Do you want to know a secret, Lor?' the girl says after a while. 'I have a plan. I have a way to escape from this.'

I look at her, curious. 'You do?'

'I'm going to kill myself,' she says.

I swallow, my throat tightening, stunned not just by what she's said but by the detached calm in her voice.

'I'm going to wait until we've merged. Then I'm going to end my life and end his at the same time. It's not like you and Amelia,' she says. 'We're not in this together. He's forcing me into it, and I need to show him, to show everyone, that it's not okay.'

I shake my head. 'You can't kill yourself.'

'Why not? I'll already be dead, in a way.' She frowns. 'You can't tell anyone this, Lor. You understand, right?'

'I have to tell someone,' I say. 'I can't let you...'

She moves closer to the mirror, smoothing her hair with the palm of her hand. 'Would it be murder?' she says. 'Or suicide? It's an interesting question, isn't it.' She tilts her head, her eyes on her reflection. 'It'll fuck up their plans if Dad dies. He's not the sort they want gone. They want to be shot of the weak people.' She looks at me, lowers her voice further. 'Think about it, Lor. You've got Alzheimer's. I'm an addict. Noah's got leukaemia. We're the misfits of society. If they find a way to successfully merge us, to get rid of our problems, then they'll do it to anyone with an ailment. Soon, only the healthy, rich ones will be left. Just like they want.'

I shake my head. It can't be true.

And yet... it makes sense. We *are* the weaker ones in the group. 'You'll have to tell me this again when I have my notebook,' I say quietly. 'When we go back into the room, make sure that I write down everything you've just told me.'

She nods.

But we're not taken back into the room. The rest of the group is waiting for us in the foyer. Amelia has my bag on her shoulder. 'Sorry.' The lady in the purple tunic checks her watch. 'We ran a little over.' She smiles. 'Well done today, everyone. Enjoy your week, and keep up your acclimatisation work. There's not long to go now.'

Amelia hands me my bag. 'How was it?' she says.

Lara answers for me. 'Creepy.'

'Really? How so?'

She shrugs. 'A room filled with mirrors is creepy. Especially when it's not your reflection looking back at you.'

'I thought they weren't going to be turning on the projections today.'

'They weren't. It was still creepy. Wasn't it, Lor?'

I nod, distracted as I rummage in my bag. I need to get my notebook out, to write down what Lara said, but by the time I've found it she's walking away. I watch as she disappears through the doors and out of the Clinic. I dig in my bag for my pen. 'Lara told me something important, Amelia,' I say. 'I need to write it down.'

'Now? Can't you do it in the van, Mum?'

'I don't want to forget. She said they want to get rid of all the weak people, and that's why we're merging.'

Amelia hushes me quickly, looking around. 'Mum, you can't say stuff like that in here.'

'Why not?'

'You just can't. Come on, let's go. I'll remember it for you. We can talk about it when we get home.'

I continue looking in my bag for my pen as I follow Amelia across the foyer and through the large doors. She stops abruptly. I bump into her. 'Amelia, why have you—' I follow her gaze, looking down the stairs to the crowd of protestors. The group is far larger than I remember.

They surge forward like a tidal wave.

I abandon my search for the pen and grip Amelia's hand. 'Ignore them,' she says. 'It's not us they're angry at. They'll shout, but they can't get to us.'

Amelia begins descending the stone steps. The van is waiting for us, guarded by security workers. My hand tightens round Amelia's, but I can't move. I stay frozen at the top of the steps, my arm outstretched. Placards wave above the sea of faces, the words large and written in red, demanding to be seen.

HUMANS, NOT EXPERIMENTS
FUCK COMBINE
REJECT THE MERGE AGENDA
BRIGHTWELL'S VISION, OUR NIGHTMARE

There's a man's face plastered across a placard, his eyes narrowed, his lips twisted into a smirk. I recognise him, his silver hair, his tanned skin. But I can't remember who he is, what role he plays. Beneath his image the words **MONSTER IN A SUIT** are scrawled in angry letters.

Faces blur in the chaos, furious voices rising over one another. The crowd's anger, even at this distance, suffocates, makes it difficult to breathe. Mitchell was in a crowd just like this, surrounded by such hatred, moments before he lost his life.

He was crushed. Trampled into the ground like dirt.

Amelia tugs at my hand, urging me forward, but I'm paralysed. My breathing is shallow, my vision blurring. My dear Mitchell. Murdered in a crowd just like this one.

Amelia has her hand on my back. She's guiding me down the steps, and somehow, I'm moving. We're halfway down when I hear her name being screamed. '*Amelia! Amelia!*' The voice is frantic. I look out into the crowd. There's a girl, about Amelia's age, jumping and waving both arms in the air, desperately trying to get her attention. 'Amelia!' she screams. 'Amelia, what the fuck are you doing?'

Amelia's got her head down, her hand pressing firmly on my back. 'Keep going, Mum,' she says. 'Please. Let's get out of here.'

'Do you know her?' I ask, but Amelia doesn't hear me. She keeps pushing me forward, increasing the pressure on my back. She speeds up, and I go with her. As we reach the bottom of the steps, I look back at the girl. She's fighting to get to the front, to get to us, but the crowd is too strong.

The wave swallows her, and I scream. 'Amelia, that girl you know, she's drowning.'

'She's fine, Mum. I don't know her. Let's get to the van. It's not safe out here with all these protestors.'

I look back at the crowd, but I can no longer see the girl.

On the drive back to the apartment, I write everything down. Amelia is silent, nibbling at the skin around her fingernails, staring out of the window. I want to ask her what just happened, who that girl was, and why the crowd was so big today. But I need to get this down before I forget.

I write everything I can remember about what Lara told me, about what she believes they're doing. I keep writing until the van stops. My eyes linger on the final line I've written:

Societal cleansing – only the rich and the healthy will be left standing.

Amelia

We're ready in Room One before the staff join us. I sit next to Mum, with Lara on her other side, the two of them talking quietly. 'The girl just seems to enjoy my company,' Mum said when I queried their newfound friendship. 'She's sweet. Angry, though. I can't say I care much for her bad language.'

Lucas sits on the other side of me, his legs swinging in anticipation. 'What do you think they'll look like?' he asks. 'We know it'll be a man, physically, right? Because they're called Rosa-Liam.'

I nod. 'The second name always belongs to the person whose body will remain,' Eliza explained our first week. 'The first name belongs to the Transfer, their incredible contribution acknowledged as an act of respect, ensuring they're not forgotten.'

'Callie said they haven't changed their appearance much,' I say. 'They still look like Liam, just with shorter hair and apparently they're in better shape than they were before.'

'Do you reckon you two will look the same after? Noah will definitely change our look. He cares about looking good and knows how to pull it off. Before he got sick, he was the guy everyone was into. Even now, they'd pick him over me. Except Ellie, obviously. I'm looking forward to it. I've never been confident. It'll be nice being the one people fancy.'

I smile. Lucas looks up to Noah the way I always imagined looking up to a sibling. I used to beg for a brother or sister, making my case at the dinner table, slipping notes under Mum and Dad's bedroom door, promising I'd be on my best behaviour forever if they just said yes. You're enough for us, they'd always say. It's better this way – you get all the love. But I was persistent, pushing until one day Mum broke down in tears. 'Are you really not happy?' she asked. I never brought it up again after that.

'Is it weird that I'm looking forward to this?' I ask. 'It feels like the first real chance we've had to find out what being a Combine is actually like.' I think of the Combines I've spoken to while filming Ceremonies, how they always turn away at my questions, their guarded eyes refusing to let me in.

'Not weird at all.' Lucas nods towards the others. Everyone looks keen to get started. Even Lara sits upright, smiling as she chats with Mum. While it's common to be in the presence of Combines nowadays, it's still a novelty to be able to question one. It's considered impolite to ask why someone merged, like forcing them to relive a painful decision.

Eliza enters with the other Support Workers. Rosa-Liam follows behind. They're tall and broad, with dark skin and short hair, faded at the temples, wearing a suit and tie in Combine green. They unbutton their jacket as they sit, the chair squeaking under their weight. I stare along with everyone else, taken aback by their presence. I'd expected a male body, but I hadn't anticipated such imposing masculinity.

Rosa-Liam's left leg begins bouncing. I watch their large thigh move quickly up and down, wondering how it must feel for Rosa to inhabit such a male body now, whether it feels different at all.

Eliza smiles at our silence. 'I know this session has been highly anticipated, and I am utterly thrilled to introduce our inaugural speaker, Rosa-Liam, who underwent the Merge five years ago. They were formerly Rosa Blackwell and Liam Abiola, and were matched by the British Pairing Company. Liam was our very own Callie's brother.'

Callie nods proudly.

'They are here today to talk to you about their experience and to answer any questions you may have. What Rosa-Liam reveals today is in the strictest confidence. This is their personal experience, and it is Rosa-Liam's right for the information they share to remain private.'

Rosa-Liam smiles, their eyes creasing, softening their features. 'Hi, everyone.' They have the rough voice of a seasoned smoker. 'It's so good to meet you all. I still remember my first speaker. I never imagined I'd become one, let alone address a group as special as yours. Let me start by saying that what you lot are doing is really brave. I was shitting myself when I went through the Preparation Period. I remember how it feels, how much you question what you're doing as the weeks go on. I hope I can put at least some of your minds at ease and alleviate a few of your worries.'

Mum's frowning, as though something's not quite making sense to her. I lean in. 'That's a Combine, Mum,' I whisper. 'We've never met them before.'

'I know that,' Mum whispers back, irritated.

We haven't had an easy morning. I found Mum crying on the sofa. She hadn't slept. She'd forgotten, momentarily, that her own mother was dead and was reliving the shock and grief all over again. 'I thought she was waiting for me to get ready for school,' she said, clutching a cushion. 'Isn't that ridiculous?'

'Like Eliza said, I formerly presented as Rosa and Liam. I was matched through the British Pairing Company – the BPC – five years ago at the Unity Clinic in Finchley. Rosa and

Liam had an exceptionally high compatibility score, just as I've been told each of you here do. I think it's incredible that you've all found matches you already know. That wasn't the case for me. I had to seek out the partnership: I went through endless tests before finding my match. It's rare to be fortunate enough to be able and willing to merge with someone you're already acquainted with, let alone someone you love.'

'Why were you so desperate to do it?' I ask. 'Was it for money?'

'No.' Rosa-Liam shakes their head. 'Money wasn't the appeal for me. I know that's why most people sign up with the BPC, but for me it was a way out of my head.' They cross their left leg over their right. 'I've always suffered from acute anxiety, and it was becoming unmanageable. There were days, often weeks, when I couldn't leave the house, couldn't enjoy any aspect of my life.'

'Who was anxious?' Annie asks. 'Rosa or Liam?'

'Rosa-Liam.'

'You both felt the same way?'

'I was suffering terribly from anxiety. I felt trapped.'

'But there were two of you,' Annie insists. 'Which one felt anxious?'

'I presented as two individuals,' Rosa-Liam says, their voice calm. 'But I am one person. I know it's difficult to understand, but I have always been one person. It's just that now I am complete.'

A silence falls over the room. We exchange glances.

'It's not instant,' Rosa-Liam continues. 'In fact, it takes a hell of a lot of work to get to this point. You'll know all about the stages by now. Stage One is easy. It's the transfer, the Merge. You're not conscious for the physical merging, so that's nothing to worry about.' They smile. 'You *will* worry about it. Of course you will. It's the part I worried about the most. Would I survive it? Would it work? Would it hurt? But the part I should have worried about was Stage Two.'

'What's Stage Two?' Mum asks.

'The Merging of Consciousness,' Rosa-Liam says. 'Adapting the brain to accept another's presence and to no longer exist as a single entity. Stage Two is where you learn to let go of your old identities and embrace your new, unified persona.'

'Gosh,' Mum gasps. 'How long does that take?'

'It took me just over seven months, but it's different for everyone.' Rosa-Liam looks at Eliza. 'I believe ten months is the average time for a Combine to be signed off?'

'Yes.' Eliza nods. 'Anywhere between six and fifteen months is normal.'

'How do you know when you're aligned?' Lara asks.

'You think in the singular,' Rosa-Liam says. 'You no longer acknowledge the fact you have two identities in one body, you just *are* one person. There's no more head-talk.'

'Head-talk?' Mum says.

'The internal dialogue,' Rosa-Liam explains. 'The constant back and forth between Rosa and Liam. At first, it felt like a crowded room in my mind, both voices competing for dominance. But over time, as we worked through Stage Two, those voices blended into one harmonious thought process. That's when I knew I was aligned, when I could think and feel as a single, complete person. I was terribly miserable before. I'm truly happy now.'

'Merging fixed your anxiety?' Lucas asks.

Rosa-Liam nods.

'It's gone?'

'Yes. It's gone.'

Lucas grins at Noah, who grins back. 'That's incredible.'

Rosa-Liam laughs. 'It's insane, is what it is. I wouldn't

believe it if it hadn't happened to me. I honestly never thought I'd be happy again.'

I stare at them, trying to gauge how they must feel, how it would feel to have my anxieties erased, to no longer wake at night haunted by the memories of Dad's death. How it would feel for Mum to no longer suffer from her confusion, no longer experience the pain of her past as if it were happening all over again. 'You don't worry about the things you used to?' I ask.

Rosa-Liam shakes their head.

'How does that work? How can your problems just disappear like that?'

Rosa-Liam's eyes soften. 'It's not that the problems disappear, it's that they are integrated into a new sense of self. The anxieties, the fears, they don't vanish, but they lose their power.' They look around the circle, at each of us hanging on their words. 'In my experience, the Combine mind is considerably more stable than that of a non-Combine.'

I glance at Mum, seeing her as she was this morning, sitting on the sofa, lost in grief, clutching that cushion. What if we could keep the good parts of ourselves and get rid of the aspects we don't like? Mum's creativity, her warmth, the way she makes even the smallest moments feel like magic – could those parts stay, while the confusion and forgotten memories slip away?

'How does the remembering work?' Jay asks. 'My memories are something I'm keen to hold on to.' He looks at Lara. 'We both are. Neither of us wants to forget. Do you have the memories from before... from both Rosa and Liam? Did you get to keep them all?'

Rosa-Liam nods. 'They're all here.'

'Do you feel as though you were there when the memories occurred?' Jay presses.

'Absolutely. I was there.'

'Not all of you,' Jay says.

'Yes. All of me.'

Lara raises her hand but doesn't wait for an invitation to speak. 'So, I'll feel like I was there for Dad's memories, even if I wasn't?' A shadow of distaste flickers across her face. 'What about when he had sex with my mum? Will I feel like I was there too? That's fucking gross.'

The question knocks me. Knowing we wouldn't be going through with it, I hadn't properly considered what merging with Mum would mean. Would I be burdened with her most private moments? The thought of experiencing her sexual memories makes my stomach churn. I don't want any part of it.

Rosa-Liam clears their throat. 'It's not quite like that. You won't feel as though you were physically there for those memories. It's more like a deep understanding of your Partner's experiences. You'll have their memories, yes, but they won't feel like your own lived moments. You can choose not to look.'

The room falls silent. Mum watches Rosa-Liam intently, as if trying to piece together who they are and why they're here. 'Is it confusing?' she asks quietly. 'Having all those memories? I struggle enough making sense of my own. I can't imagine adding someone else's into the mix. I have... I have Alzheimer's, you see.'

Rosa-Liam offers a reassuring smile. 'It'll be clearer than ever for you, Laurie. Just as my anxiety was lifted, I'm certain your confusion will ease as well.'

As Rosa-Liam speaks, I find myself picturing a future where Mum is free from the fog of Alzheimer's, where we could work together to recall her memories, and she could live without the constant weight of confusion.

I look at her, hunched over her notebook. Her pen moves

quickly, her face tight with concentration as she races to capture a thought before it slips away.

Could I really bring her back? Could I take her dementia from her, just as Rosa-Liam's anxiety was taken? The possibility feels both hopeful and terrifying. All I have to do is decide. If Mum were her old self again, fully able to grasp what merging meant, what would she want? Would she choose for us to go through with this, to spend the rest of our lives together? Or would she want me to fight?

For the first time, I wonder if merging could actually be the answer.

Not just for her, but for us.

Laurie

Mary and I have spent so much of our lives sitting in camping chairs. She moved to London as soon as she was old enough to leave home, and camping chairs were the first thing she bought, one for her and one for me. For a long time, they were her only items of furniture, aside from the air-mattress her parents had begrudgingly let her take. Every weekend, I'd catch the train to London, and we'd haul the chairs to Primrose Hill. We'd spend the day drinking warm cans of beer, speculating about our futures, laughing about nothing.

When the sun set, we'd fold the chairs and carry them home.

Sometimes we discussed the possibility of her buying more furniture or framing the art we'd taped up, but it was only ever make-believe. Mary didn't need anything else. The day Stuart, who later became her husband, moved in and insisted on decorating, Mary and I watched as he nailed cheap prints to the walls, lurid landscapes and splashy street art, ruining her home with his 'vision'.

Today, we've set up on the path in front of St Michael's. Mary's propped the small collapsible table between our chairs and set out paintboxes, brushes, a roll of paper towel and a jar of water. No easels today. We've opted for our sketchbooks, balanced on our knees.

The church's brick is warm and uneven, its edges softened, rounded by time. Arched stained-glass windows scatter fractured colours onto the path, shifting as the sunlight moves.

I dip my brush in the water and let the paint bloom across the page in soft, translucent waves. I layer ochre and sienna. The colours bleed together, creating a hazy background that mirrors the texture of the church bricks. As I work, I wonder what's happening inside, beyond the glass. I picture someone kneeling in a pew, their hands clasped tightly, pleading with God to hear them. To help. The faint murmurs of their prayer rising to the vaulted ceiling.

For two years following Mitchell's death, I attended church every Sunday. After my childhood, I never thought I'd set foot in a church again, but I found myself needing God. I needed the insistence of the congregation that Mitchell was, without a doubt, spending eternity with Him in heaven.

I pause to apply suncream, watching as Mary blends a little crimson into the pale blue wash of the sky. She has a distinct style, yet it has become increasingly similar to my own. Our recent paintings could easily be muddled up. In a way, I suppose we're merging. How could we not, after fifty years of painting together?

'It's getting worse, Mary,' I say, returning the suncream to my bag.

'Tell me about it.' She frowns at her sketchbook. 'My sky is irrecoverably muddy.'

'Not my painting, my brain.'

Mary looks up, her paintbrush hovering above her sketchbook.

'I have these moments of blankness where it's like part of my brain has been erased.'

'What did the doctor say last week at your check-up? Amelia mentioned new medication.'

I frown. 'I remember the appointment, but I can't really...'

I shake my head. 'See what I mean? It's there – the memory – but I can't get at it. I know I went. And afterwards I know we went to a café. The one in the bookshop by the clock tower. But I can't remember what happened at the doctors, or what was said. That part's been rubbed out. I had something tasty… something warm. At the café, I mean.' I tap my foot, trying to bring the memory into focus. What was it I ate? I click my fingers when it finally comes to me. 'I had a freshly baked scone, Mary.'

She nods.

'Mary?'

'Yes?'

'I don't want Amelia to waste her life worrying about me.'

'She's your daughter, Lor. Of course she's going to worry about you.'

'I don't want her to be like me, like I was.'

Mary plunges her paintbrush into the water, darkening it to a deep blue as she swirls her brush clean. 'Your mother was so lucky to have you.'

'Nothing about my mother was lucky.'

Mary rips off a sheet of paper towel and begins drying her brush. 'How is the merging preparation going, Lor?'

'Fine, I think.' I watch as the paper towel turns translucent. 'It's difficult for me to remember. So much happens in the sessions, so many people talk about complicated things. All the information just blurs together.'

'Are you using your notebook?'

'Oh, yes. Good idea.' I reach into my handbag. The notebook already looks worn, despite my only having had it for a couple of months. The leather cover is faded and creased and there's an ink stain in the corner. I turn to my most recent notes.

<u>Questions for Saturday's interview:</u>
PREPARE ANSWERS THIS WEEK

1. Can you tell me about your earliest childhood memories?

2. How would you describe your relationship with your family during your formative years?

3. Can you recall any specific challenges or traumas from your childhood that may have had a lasting impact on you?

4. How would you describe your relationship with your parents?

5. Are there positive or negative memories associated with specific places from your past?

6. Can you share any experiences that shaped your identity or sense of self during adolescence?

7. Are there specific memories that you find particularly vivid or emotionally charged?

8. How would you describe your romantic relationships throughout different life stages?

9. Are there any recurring themes or patterns in your memories that you've noticed over time?

10. Are there specific memories that you feel have had a lasting impact on your emotional well-being?

Mary looks at me expectantly. 'Well?'

'Well, what?' I get a pencil from my bag and start to scribble down answers.

'Did it help?'

'Did what help, Mary? Sorry, I can't talk right now. There's something I've got to get sorted.' I focus on working my way through the questions as Mary continues painting. She's uncharacteristically quiet.

'Are you okay?' I ask once I've finished.

'I am okay, Lor. It's just... I find it hard when I think about what you and Amelia are doing. I know it's the modern world and I need to get used to it. And I love Amelia for being so intent on saving your memories. It just... it concerns me, that's all. You know it does.'

I'm unsure if I've been in this room before. The weeks are passing so quickly that it's increasingly difficult to remember what I've done. Something about the room feels familiar, and yet I'm not entirely sure what it's used for. The walls are an icy blue, and a small walnut desk sits against the far wall. On the shelf beside me are framed photographs of teenage girls holding trophies. They're fair-haired and wearing football kits streaked with mud. Mitchell always hoped Amelia would grow to take an interest in football, that she'd come round to the notion of supporting West Ham one day.

Amelia and I are sitting on brown leather armchairs opposite a man on a matching sofa. *Nathan, Support Worker.* He scratches at a mark on the armrest as he talks. Amelia listens intently, nodding along.

I must not have been in this room before. I like to think I'd remember the large oil painting on the wall behind the sofa. It's of Bangkok, before the temples were submerged. In the painting, a woman sits in front of a temple, her legs crossed, her feet bare. Her expression is joyful, as though she's just seen someone she loves. I turn to a new page in my notebook and write a large title. _Painting of Bangkok._ I underline it twice. It seems important, somehow.

'Laurie?' the man says. 'Are you following along?'

I look up from my page, blinking. I'd not realised I was supposed to be listening.

'The sessions are really taking a toll on Mum,' Amelia says, her hand finding my knee. 'She's started falling asleep as soon as we get home. I know there's nothing abnormal about being tired after a long day, but it's strange seeing Mum so tired. She's never tired. Not like this.' She lifts her hand from my knee. 'When Mum's tired, Nathan, she zones out. So she might appear to be more forgetful than she actually is.'

I eye Amelia. I can always tell when she's lying – the subtle shift in her voice, a change in inflection that's given her away since she was a child. Like that Christmas when she insisted, far too sweetly, that she hadn't peeked at her presents. I remember how she tore into the wrapping paper with just a touch too much enthusiasm, and the exaggerated gasp of surprise over the new water bottle. 'I had no idea,' she said, her voice too high-pitched to be genuine, hugging the bottle like it was a doll. 'This is just what I wanted.'

If I were really exhausted, like Amelia's saying, wouldn't we have discussed it? She's been so good at keeping track of my lifestyle choices and how they correlate to the disease. Perhaps tiredness is something we have spoken about. I can't recall. I flick back through the notebook, searching for any mention of sleep.

Skimming the pages is overwhelming. There's so much in there that I know, but also a great deal that I don't remember. Certain words stand out. Nathan – this man – is in here a lot.

'Laurie?' Nathan says. His tone tells me this isn't the first time he's said my name.

'Sorry.' I look up from my notes. 'Yes?'

'I asked if there was anything you're especially worried about? Amelia was just speaking about the fear she has of letting you down if the Merge fails.'

I look at Amelia. She's staring at her lap, a crease between her eyebrows that I haven't noticed before. I wonder what I've done to upset her this time. I'm always getting it wrong, always making her storm off and slam her bedroom door. Parenting is so difficult. We never seem to get it right.

'Is there anything specific you're worried about, Laurie?'

'I worry about a lot of things,' I say. 'I worry about all of this merging nonsense.'

'Nonsense?' Nathan repeats, his eyebrows raised. 'What in particular are you worrying about?'

'Well, I'm glad you've asked, actually.' I start searching for the list of questions I've written. I remember writing them. I flick through the pages. The sheer volume of information in my notebook is astonishing. I read as I search. There's so much in there that I recognise, but also a great deal that I don't remember. Nathan – this man – is in here a lot.

'Mum,' Amelia says gently, 'can I help you find what you're looking for?'

I shake my head. 'I'll find it, Amelia. Just be patient with me.'

I stop flicking when I come across a note I've underlined repeatedly:

<u>Combine has a hidden agenda!</u>

'What is Combine's hidden agenda?' I ask, holding the notebook up. 'I have it written down here, you see.' I show Amelia the page, and she reads over my scribbles.

'Hidden agenda?' Nathan repeats. 'Who told you that Combine has a hidden agenda, Laurie?'

'Lara,' Amelia says dryly. 'All these notes are about a conversation you had with Lara, Mum. She doesn't want to be here doing any of this, remember? She's not the most trustworthy source of information.'

Nathan leans forward slightly. 'Amelia's right, Laurie. It's important to consider the source of our information. Lara's perspective is valid, but it's one of many. I wouldn't advise going to her for clarification on the merging process. The only agenda Combine has is to prevent the deterioration of humanity and, all being well, rid the world of currently incurable diseases.'

I eye the microphone on Nathan's collar. 'Why are you wearing that?'

'For the recordings.' He smiles. 'You're wearing one, too. So is Amelia.'

I glance down, expecting him to be wrong. But there it is – small, black, clipped neatly to the neck of my dress. A microphone. I frown. How long has it been there? How much has it heard?

'It's nothing to worry about, Mum. It's to help you, to help us both. We can listen back to the recordings, remember? You've done lots of these interviews, Mum. You spent an hour with Nathan earlier, just the two of you. Don't you remember?'

I shake my head.

'Not to worry,' Nathan says. 'Perhaps I'll play you a recording once we're done here. I'll ensure you're alone, so Amelia doesn't hear.'

'I don't mind Amelia hearing,' I say. 'What are these recordings?'

'They're your innermost thoughts and feelings, any secrets you're keeping from Amelia. You sit with me as you listen back to them. Do you remember any of this?'

I shake my head again.

Nathan smiles kindly. 'Well, we'll make sure you have some time to listen later. The more you listen, the easier it becomes to share your deepest thoughts. The more you confront the parts of yourself you wish to keep hidden, the easier it will become to share yourself freely with your Partner. Do you understand?'

I nod, though I don't understand.

'Is there anything you want to talk about, Laurie? Any feelings you have that you'd like to share with Amelia?'

I look at her, and she nods encouragingly. 'Go on, Mum. Share with me. I'll be finding out all your secrets in a few weeks anyway. You may as well tell me some of them.'

'Start with something simple,' Nathan says. 'Why don't you tell Amelia something from your past, something that she doesn't know about?'

'Something from my...'

I remember. I remember, with sudden clarity, the microphone recording my words, the drip, drip, drip of my deepest secrets disappearing into it as I looked at the painting of Bangkok. I know what Nathan and I talked about. I know what he wants me to tell Amelia. But I don't know if I can.

'Go on, Lor,' he says gently. 'Being honest with Amelia will make everything easier when you merge.'

I look at her.

'Why don't you tell her about your feelings regarding marriage?' Nathan's watching me as though he thinks I'm about to shatter. 'We spoke about that earlier, Lor, do you remember?'

I nod, though I can't recall the specifics of how we got onto the topic. I do remember discussing marriage, confiding in him about the anxieties that have plagued me for years. I know it's irrational, and I know the chances of Albie and Amelia marrying are slim, but the worry has been a constant companion. Many sleepless nights have been spent fretting over the father-of-the-bride speech, dreading the father-daughter dance.

'Go on, Mum,' Amelia says gently. 'Tell me.'

I close my eyes, the memories pressing against my lids. 'I always found the thought of my wedding so painful,' I say finally. 'Until I met your father, I dreaded getting married.'

Amelia frowns. 'But you're obsessed with weddings and babies, and all that traditional crap. Why would you dread it?'

'I didn't want to get married without my mother.' My voice breaks. 'I didn't even want to fall in love without her being there to witness it. It still hurts me, you know, that she never saw me in love, that she never met Mitch. Never met you. The loves of my life never once laid eyes on each other, not beyond the photographs I showed your father when I was missing her so terribly.'

'Why don't you ever talk about her?'

Nathan gives me a small nod of encouragement.

'My mother had a difficult life, Amelia. A life filled with pain and fear.'

She waits.

I take a deep breath, my fingers gathering the fabric of my dress, twisting it beneath my hands. 'My stepfather, Tony, he...' I bite my lip, willing myself not to cry, not to let the old wounds bleed anew. 'He would hit her, Amelia. He drove her to drink, and then he assaulted her for it.'

Amelia looks at her lap, her hair falling forward, obscuring her expression.

'I spent my childhood looking out for her, trying to keep her safe. And I didn't manage it, Amelia. I never... I couldn't...'

I can't say any more. I untwist my dress, smoothing the fabric over my lap. My mind drifts to the bathtub. The slow drip of my mother's blood pooling on the tiled floor.

'Oh, Mum,' she whispers. 'I'm so sorry. Did he... Was his violence only directed at your mum? Or did he ever...'

I shake my head. 'Only twice. And only when I got between them. He never came after me. Never more than holding my arm too tightly or attacking me with his words. It was my mother he wanted to hurt, not me.'

Amelia is silent for a while. Then, quietly, 'What happened to him?'

'He passed away a year before your father did. It was Mitch who broke the news to me. I can't recall how he found out.' I swallow, bracing myself. 'There's something else, Amelia.'

She doesn't need this now, not after what I've just told her. But now that I've started, the words pour out, unstoppable. 'Your father and I, we had – trouble – before you.' My voice falters, the memories as clear as they ever were. The cramps. The bleeding. The fractured trust in my body. 'I had pregnancies, multiple, that didn't last. We tried, and tried, refused to give up hope. Then, it finally happened. A miracle. Harrison.'

Amelia's face stills, her brows drawn together.

'Harrison was born three weeks premature,' I continue, my voice wavering. 'With a poor immune system. Weak lungs. Nothing fatal, the doctors said, just not as strong as we'd hoped. They told us he'd grow, get stronger. But he didn't.'

Her lips part, her head shaking slightly. My little girl, my Amelia, hearing a story that doesn't make sense. 'Who...?'

'Harrison,' I whisper. 'Your brother. He died when he was only two.'

Her confusion fractures into something sharper.

'What the fuck? I had a brother?'

I nod, my throat tightening. 'It's why your father was hellbent on protesting, why he dedicated his life to demanding solutions for the pollution that infected Harrison's lungs. He coped by fighting against the thing that killed his son.' I press my hand to my eyes, trying to stem the tears. 'I don't know how I coped. I'm not sure I did.'

Amelia stares at me, her mouth open. 'I... I don't...'

'We swore we'd not go through it again, that we'd not try for another baby. We couldn't stand the idea of suffering that heartache again. But, ten years later, the most remarkable thing happened. I fell pregnant with you, Amelia.'

Amelia

I shake my head, unable to process it.

Mum nods, wiping her eyes.

I turn to Nathan. He nods too. He knew. He knew about my brother. Mum told him, and not me. 'Why the fuck did you never tell me any of this?'

Mum flinches. 'You were so little,' she says quietly, her eyes fixed on her notebook. 'It's not an easy or appropriate conversation to have with a young child. A toddler dying is not something a child should have to think about.'

'I've not been a child in years,' I say, my voice trembling.

She keeps staring at the pages. 'We were going to tell you. We almost told you so many times. But you're such a worrier, so much like your father. We didn't want to darken your world. Then Mitch died. And I… Without him, I couldn't do it. I just couldn't.'

The room seems to tilt. A ship caught in a storm. I clutch my chair. 'So that's why Dad protested? Why he never missed a rally?'

Mum looks at me. 'He devoted his life to ensuring no other child would die like Harrison did.'

Harrison. My brother.

I collapse inward, suddenly racked with grief for the brother I never knew, the brother who was kept from me. I think of Dad, how little he slept, how often I'd catch him staring into space, lost in his sorrow. I never understood why he cared so much, why he marched for hours in the rain until his feet blistered and his voice went raw.

If I'd known, if they'd told me, I'd have done more. I'd have helped. I'd have been there the day Dad died.

'Now do you understand why I don't want to do this?' Mum's voice is sharp, as though I'm the one who's been keeping secrets. 'I don't want to pass all this trauma on to you, Amelia. I have a lifetime of it. I've done everything in my power to protect you, to keep you from suffering the way I did. I refuse to let you take it on. I refuse to burden you with it.'

'Did Dad know that I loved him?'

She says nothing.

The silence presses on my chest until I can hardly breathe.

'I know he knew when I was younger, but the day he died – do you think he knew that I loved him then? When I refused to go with him to the protest? I... I told him I hated him. It's the last thing he ever heard me say.'

But Mum doesn't reply. She frowns, looking around. When she notices me watching her, she leans in close. 'Aren't there normally more people here?'

I shake my head, desperate. She can't do this now. She can't leave me like this.

'This is a private session,' Nathan says calmly. 'For you and Amelia. Everyone else is with their designated Support Workers. You're here with me because I'm going to be your Support Worker once you've merged, remember? This is your private session, Laurie.'

Mum's eyes drift around the room, lost, before landing on me again. She frowns. 'This is what I don't like about these meetings. You always get upset.' She folds her arms and turns to Nathan. 'I don't think it's appropriate for children to be here. How much longer are we expected to stay? Everyone else seems to have gone home.'

Nathan addresses me. 'What would you like to do? Have a break and resume later? Or do you think you'd best get Laurie home?'

Mum's eyes fix on me, her brow still furrowed. 'What are you doing here, Amelia? You really shouldn't come to these meetings. They're awfully sad. No place for a child. I shouldn't be here, either. But I don't like leaving my mother alone.' She looks around the room. 'Where is she?'

'Come on.' I stand. 'Let's go home.'

'What time is it?'

'Two thirty.'

'Good.' Mum nods. 'We've still got plenty of time. Come on then, Amelia. Let's get you home before he realises we're missing.'

Laurie

Mary and I made sure we painted this afternoon. We're sitting in the garden, our easels in front of us, sharing a flask of tea.

I haven't managed to maintain the garden the way Mitchell would have liked. The flowerbeds are overgrown, weeds sprouting between the plants. I've no real idea what I've got growing. I keep meaning to ask Amelia to help me tidy the beds, but I never remember to mention it. I look around for Mitchell's olive tree. It's not here. I stand up, searching for the bird table, the greenhouse. 'This isn't my garden,' I tell Mary. 'Whose garden are we in?'

'The community garden, Lor. For your block.' She smiles. 'Your garden was much nicer than this one. You looked after it so well once Mitch passed. Everything seemed to flourish under your care.' She opens the paintbox we've set up on the little collapsible table between our camping chairs. The blue, white and red are almost out. We always use every bit of paint before we restock. 'I can't believe this is it, Lor. Our last time painting together.'

I pick up the flask and pour the tea carefully into our mugs. 'I'll still be able to paint afterwards. It's not really the last time.'

She takes her mug. 'You're really doing it? You know, I didn't think you would. At least, I hoped you wouldn't.'

I nod. 'Neither did I. But it's what Amelia wants. And all I want is for her to be happy.'

Mary sets her mug down at her feet. 'And you truly believe that merging will make her happy? You don't think she'll live to regret her decision?'

'I don't know,' I say honestly. 'But I'm exhausted, Mary. I can't keep arguing with her. It's making us both miserable. If I back out and refuse to merge, I don't think she'll ever forgive me. And I'm not sure I'll forgive myself either. I'll just get worse, and she'll end up spending the rest of my life caring for me, all because I was too afraid to go through with it.'

Mary dips her paintbrush into the burnt umber and begins making shadows on the paper. 'How will I know I'm speaking to you? How will I know that you're there and it's not just Amelia?'

'I think you'll just know.'

She shakes her head. 'That's not good enough. I want evidence that you're the one listening to me, that I'm not only talking to Amelia. How about a codeword? You'll say it to me, and I'll know you're the one speaking.'

I raise my eyebrows as I begin painting. 'There's one flaw to your plan.' I tickle what's left of the vermillion with my brush. 'I'll have to remember the code.'

'Won't Amelia be able to remember for you? Isn't that the point?'

'I suppose so.'

She sighs. 'It's all so strange and unnatural, Lor. I can't understand how it all works. Doesn't the whole thing terrify you?'

'Of course it does.'

'So why do it? Why not let nature take its course, let your Alzheimer's progress.' Her eyes fill with tears. 'It's terrible, but it happens. Millions of people live with Alzheimer's, Lor. I'm certain you still have so many good years ahead of you. You just have to keep going.'

'So, what, I keep going until... Until the good years are over?'

Mary nods. 'Until the good years are over.'

I swirl my brush in the jar of water. 'I'm not sure I have many good years left in me, Mary. I'm increasingly bad at retaining information, remembering what's been said. There's so much to all of this merging that I still don't understand, even after these months of preparation. Isn't that ridiculous?'

'Not at all ridiculous.'

'I can't seem to keep hold of the facts. I couldn't tell you the first thing about it without reading my notes. And even then, it's so difficult to make sense of.'

'Of course it is. This whole thing is difficult to make sense of. Oh, come here.' Mary puts her paintbrush down and leans over to hug me tightly. 'I love you, Lor,' she says. 'No matter what.'

'You must think I'm pathetic.'

'Anything but,' she whispers. 'You silly sod.'

I smile. 'I like that – for our codeword, *silly sod.*'

She releases me and pulls her sketchbook from her bag, flipping through it until she finds a blank page. She tears it out, writes *SILLY SOD* in bold letters, folds the paper in half and hands it to me. 'So, when I ask for proof you're there, listening to me, you'll call me a silly sod. Promise?'

I nod.

'Good. Amelia would never use that phrase.'

I slip the paper into my bag, and we get back to painting. We paint until Mary has to leave for work. She hugs me. 'You're Committing tomorrow, Lor,' she says quietly. 'Talk to Amelia. Make sure you understand completely what you're getting yourself into.'

I hold her tightly. 'I will,' I say. 'I will, Mary.'

Albie has come to spend his last day with Amelia. They're in her bedroom. I can hear his soothing voice as he comforts her. I've been sitting at the dining room table for hours, slowly working my way through my notebook. There's so much here. So many entries I can't recall writing. I've got a highlighter, and I've been scoring anything that concerns me in yellow.

When I finish reading the latest entry, I turn back to the beginning. I take a pen and a piece of paper, and I start writing a list of all the things I've highlighted.

Under 18s have no choice
Long-term consequences of merging unknown
Reproductive rights of Combines not yet decided
Violation of human dignity!
Societal cleansing
<u>*Combine has a hidden agenda!*</u>
Validity of consent?
Huge pressure being applied to Participants – are they making an informed decision?
Potential psychological trauma
Loss of autonomy
Over 90% of existing relationships break down post-Merge – Albie and Amelia?!

I glance at the bedroom door. They're still in there. Lately, the way they've been acting – it's odd. I can't shake the feeling that I've barely seen Albie. Or maybe I have, and I'm just not remembering. But something isn't right. That uneasy feeling creeps in again.

I keep going, flicking through the pages for the scores of yellow. There, in bold, highlighted and underlined multiple times in different colours, is a note. The ink stands out – red, blue, green, black. Demanding to be heard:

<u>**LARA PLANS TO COMMIT SUICIDE ONCE MERGED**</u>

I read it again. And again. I blink incessantly, hoping my eyes are playing tricks on me. But the words remain, refusing to distort into something less horrifying.

This is clearly a note I've come back to again and again. I stare at it. How many times must I have read this page? How could I have forgotten this – even for a moment?

I hurry to Amelia's bedroom before I can forget again, the notebook clutched tightly in my hand. I go to knock but hesitate as I hear voices on the other side. My hand falters mid-air. Amelia and Albie are arguing, their tones low and urgent.

'Why can't you accept that I've changed my mind?'

What's Amelia changed her mind about? Merging?

I let out a long breath. Maybe she doesn't want this. Maybe she's feeling the same way I am. Maybe she's decided this is wrong after all.

Albie's voice slices through the door. 'You've lost your fucking mind, not changed it. The Merge is bullshit, Amelia. You know it is.'

'I *thought* it was, Albie. I don't anymore.'

I frown, the familiar sense of confusion setting in.

'So, you support this experiment? You think that forcing people to give up their bodies, their autonomy, is the solution?'

'Obviously not. But, Albie, I'm serious. I *want* to do this. All the Combines I've met are so happy. Honestly, every single one of them says that their life now is so much better than it was before as a non-Combine.'

My stomach sinks. She does want this. She wants to merge. But she didn't before…

'You mean the speakers? The ones *hired* by Combine, vetted before they speak to you?'

There's a pause. Then, 'I know what you're insinuating, but you can't deny that life as a Combine is a shitload easier.'

Albie's voice is so quiet that I struggle to hear it. 'How the fuck have they done this? How have they convinced you merging is a good thing?'

'By providing me with the truth, with the facts. Not fucking conspiracy theories.'

'Lor doesn't even want to merge. You know how much she loves you. She's going along with this because she thinks it's what you want.'

'It *is* what I want.'

'No, it fucking isn't!' he shouts.

She tries to hush him, but it doesn't work.

'You're in this to expose them, Amelia. Stop lying to me.'

There's a silence. I press my ear to the door, straining to catch any sound, but no one speaks. The notebook in my hand feels heavier. I glance at the words again. So many colours.

<u>LARA PLANS TO COMMIT SUICIDE ONCE MERGED</u>.

Finally, Amelia speaks, her voice subdued. 'Fine. That's how it started. I *was* trying to expose them. But I'm not anymore, Albs. I'm honestly not.'

'It's why you've been filming, isn't it? Why you started shooting Commitment Ceremonies in the first place?'

I frown. Amelia has filmed Ceremonies for years. I've been helping her for years. She's never alluded to doing anything with the footage beyond creating those beautiful films.

But she's admitting it. 'Yes,' she says. 'I started making a film. I was trying to show what terrible things they do to manipulate Participants into merging. But it was all for nothing, Albs. Because there's nothing malicious about it. They just support you, just help you. You just sit in circles and talk. It's completely innocent.'

'Why didn't you tell me about the film?'

'I couldn't risk it getting out. You've already been arrested twice. I didn't want to put you in danger.'

My heart lurches. Albie's been arrested? Twice? What was he arrested for?

A tangle of confusion and concern knots in my stomach.

'So, what? You're going to delete years of footage? Throw it away because you quite enjoyed the group fucking therapy sessions with people who believe they have no choice but to merge?'

Their argument continues, but I'm no longer listening. I think of all the times I've walked past Amelia's bedroom and heard her talking to herself. She always sounded so angry, so miserable. The camera on the tripod, set up with the light. I'd catch her sometimes, standing in front of it, and she'd jump. Embarrassed, I presumed, by her vanity.

But it wasn't vanity. It was a project. She wasn't ever talking to herself; she was talking to the camera. She didn't plan on merging with me to save my memories. She's far too intelligent to give up her mind like that. Amelia was in this to expose the company – the one she knew her father would have detested. 'Dad would be rolling in his grave,' she always says. 'Imagine how sickened he'd be by the state of the world.'

She was standing up against it. She was putting herself on the line.

I close my eyes. Finally, I understand. Finally, it all makes sense.

'Lor?'

I jump, opening my eyes. Albie stands in front of me. Amelia peers out from behind him, her eyes on the notebook still in my hand, my thumb tucked between the pages of Lara's suicidal confession.

'Amelia…' My voice breaks. 'I don't want to do this.'

She stares.

I show her the words, bold and stark on the page. 'Please, Amelia. I don't want to merge.'

Amelia

I turn to inspect my profile in the mirror. The green silk dress I'm wearing is low-cut, with puffed sleeves trimmed in antique-style lace. The silk hangs, light as air, no curves left for it to cling to. The neckline accentuates the flatness of my chest, that plane of pale skin where my cleavage once was. I knew I was getting smaller. I haven't had much of an appetite since we were accepted onto the trial. But I hadn't realised just how much my body had changed until now.

'Here,' Nathan said when he handed me the dress wrapped in delicate cream tissue paper. 'I thought you should have something special to wear under your ceremonial robes.'

I shook my head. 'Nathan, you really didn't need to. I already have a perfectly good dress I can wear.'

'This one's special,' he said. 'Jules helped me pick it out. I'm no fashion expert, but Jules has always had a good eye. Even the girls trust her taste. She said it was one of the most beautiful dresses she'd ever seen.'

'You really didn't have to—'

'I wanted to.' He smiled. 'It's going to be a real adventure, isn't it?'

My purple robe hangs on the clothes rail beside Mum's. It feels strange, wearing this dress, putting on the robes, just to say goodbye.

I was up all night. I sat with Mum and Albie for hours,

talking everything through. It was the moment I'd envisioned when I first signed up for the Preparation Period; my plan all along had been to make it to the end and for Mum to refuse at the last minute. It was what I'd orchestrated, what I'd depended on.

And yet, when the moment finally came, I was disappointed. Devastated.

I struggled to hold back tears as Mum, her hand firmly in mine, read out the list she'd compiled: every reason she felt uneasy about Combine, every fear she had about merging. Everything she said made sense. Every word was true. But even as her logic unfolded, all I could think about was what it would mean for us.

Mum's Alzheimer's wouldn't improve; I couldn't save her mind from slipping away.

'Are you sure?' The question caught in my throat. 'Are you absolutely sure? Even if it means not getting better?' I searched her face for some flicker of doubt, barely whispering the next question: 'Even if it means forgetting me?'

She answered with such calm certainty, her voice so steady and clear, that there was no room left for hope. 'I'm sure, Amelia. I don't want to do this. I don't want to merge with you.'

Albie, who had been silent until then, finally spoke. 'So, when do you tell them? Can we call now?' He checked his watch; it was well past midnight.

'No,' I said quietly. 'I'll call Nathan in the morning.'

Mum went to bed shortly after, and Albie prepared to leave. At the door, he kissed me – just once. 'I love you, Mills,' he said.

I nodded and watched as he turned and walked away.

I stayed up, reading Mum's notebook from cover to cover, folding the corners of the pages that held anything useful, insights she'd recorded. It struck me then: Mum had been doing my job all along. She'd remained vigilant, sceptical, cataloguing every troubling detail, quietly conducting her own investigation, right up to the very end.

Then I came across the line about Lara's suicidal intention.

I stared at the page, remembering the night Mum first mentioned it, an ordinary weekday evening. She'd been reading through her notes in the other room, and when she came into the lounge she was pacing, her movements frantic. 'It's societal cleansing, Amelia,' she said. 'They're going to kill all the weak. No one can stop it.'

She rushed out and returned moments later with her notebook in hand. She sat beside me on the sofa, flipping frantically through the pages.

That's when I saw it – bold, written in capitals, underlined so many times. A sentence that looked as if it had been carved into the paper.

'Mum?' I asked, pointing at the words. 'What's this…'

Her hands flew to her mouth, her eyes wide with sudden panic. 'Oh, god. Amelia. That poor girl. She's…' Her voice faltered. 'She's going to have a bath, and then… She's… Oh, how awful, Amelia. To slit your wrists like that.'

Mum crumpled, sobbing into my shoulder, her whole body shaking. I held her close, trying to comfort her, but I couldn't make sense of what she was saying.

I flipped through the notebook to check the date Mum had written the entry. It was from weeks earlier. I stared at it. 'Why didn't you tell me this before, Mum? Why haven't you mentioned it?'

I continued to comfort her, promising everything would be alright. We went to Eliza first thing on Saturday morning. We waited outside Room One before the session began. I expected shock, urgency – something – but when Mum shared what was in the notebook, Eliza just nodded sadly, as though she'd been expecting it.

Mum opened the page, pointing to the line she'd written. Eliza glanced at it briefly, then nodded again, her expression calm, almost resigned. 'Lara will come to terms with the Merge,' she said quietly. 'That's precisely why we have these months of preparation. Her fears are not unusual. She'll find her way through. Everyone does, eventually.'

'But don't you have a duty of care?' I whispered. Lara was just beyond the door. 'If someone – a *child* – is so desperately opposed to this, shouldn't they be listened to?'

Mum thrust the notebook at Eliza again. 'She wants to die. She's suicidal. Look, it's written here.'

'She's afraid,' Eliza said calmly. 'She's emotional, Laurie.'

'She told me she—'

'Laurie, I've been doing this for years. Lara isn't the first to make such claims. These things never come to fruition. It's a cry for help, nothing more.'

I stared at her, stunned by the casual dismissal. 'Then you should help.'

'I am helping,' Eliza said, her voice softening. She offered Mum a faint smile. 'Laurie, you've brought this to my attention twice already. Don't you remember?'

I blinked, caught off guard. Mum had spoken to Eliza about this before?

'I have?'

'Yes. And we discussed it at length both times.'

Mum's face twisted. 'I don't—'

'Lara is being well supported. She was before you raised this concern, and she continues to be now. We've spoken with Lara at great length, and she's admitted to exaggerating her fears. She feels embarrassed by her dramatic claims.' Eliza paused, cleared her throat. 'Lara told you herself that she has no intention of harming herself. Don't you remember? In my office? She's afraid, yes, but that's all. And she has every right to be. Everyone's waiting. Let's head inside. I appreciate how much you care about Lara. Looking out for one another will be so important once you're all in The Village.'

That was weeks ago. We'd raised the concern and been dismissed. Ignored. I wasn't going to let that happen again. I took the notebook into my room, turned on my computer and started dragging clips onto a timeline, piecing together what would become the point of our last three months: a clear indictment of Combine. I photographed Mum's notes and archived them safely on the Mac. Each page felt more significant now, not just memories and useful notes, but evidence that needed to be preserved.

I integrated the photographs into the edit, layering them over the interviews I'd conducted prior to Commitment Ceremonies. Tearful confessions played out on screen, the voices of Partners worn down by financial burdens, by circumstances that offered no other way out. 'It's alright,' a woman said, her voice weak. 'At least this way, we keep on going.' Others spoke excitedly about the futures they believed the Merge would secure for them, the benefits, the promises of stability. Of all the Partners I interviewed, only one spoke purely of love, his calm, peaceful voice out of place among the others. 'I get to exist inside her,' he said. 'What a dream.'

I sorted through the clips of Lara, countless shots of her looking miserable, arguing with Jay, sitting alone with her head in her hands. It was there for everyone to see: this child wanted anything but to go through with this.

I knew what we had to do. We'd go to the Clinic in the morning. I'd bring my camera and find some time to talk to Lara, to explain everything. Not just to her, but to all of them. We had to be honest with our friends about our concerns, about the ethical questions Mum's notes raised. If they still chose to go ahead with the Merge, we'd stand by them. We'd attend their Ceremony, sit in their Circle of Support. But we wouldn't join them on the other side.

Once I had a recording of Lara talking about how she felt, especially when she made that statement to Mum, I'd put together the first draft of the video. Then I'd show Albie. We'd figure out how to release it, when to make it public. This wasn't just a series of disjointed clips anymore; it was a cohesive narrative, a story with purpose. A warning to anyone ready to listen.

I broke the news to Nathan this morning. 'What do you mean you're backing out?' His voice, coming through the phone, carried an amused disbelief. 'This is just last-minute nerves, Amelia. Everyone goes through it.'

'It's not nerves,' I said, my grip tightening round the phone. 'We don't want to do it.'

There was a pause, a long one. When he spoke again, his tone was different, crushed, almost pleading. 'But all those months of preparation… You're not thinking straight, Amelia. If it's anxiety, I can prescribe something, a tablet to—'

'We want to see the others before the Ceremony, Nathan. We want to say goodbye.'

Amelia

It was Eliza who insisted we put on our ceremonial robes and do our hair and makeup. 'It would be such a shame if you had a rethink and weren't prepared,' she said, walking us to our room. 'We don't want you to miss out because of a bad case of cold feet. Go and get ready, and then see how you feel once you're with the others.'

'What room is Lara in?' I asked. 'I'd like to check on her before the Ceremony.'

Eliza smiled. 'That's thoughtful of you, Amelia, but there's no need. You'll see her soon. Everyone will gather in Room One before the Ceremony begins.' She opened the door. 'Here we are. Everything you need – shoes, robes, ribbons – is in here.'

The robes are identical, deep purple and floor length. I slip mine on over my dress and begin sorting out the ribbon, cutting it to the correct length. Mum's gone somewhere. She slipped out the room without me noticing. I peered down the corridor when I realised she was missing, but she was nowhere to be seen. A sickening thought takes hold: what if she's with Eliza or Nathan right now, spilling the details of my video, of what I plan to do once we've said our goodbyes? If she tells them, everything falls apart. I braid the first strand into my hair, my hands trembling, the ribbon almost too slippery to hold.

Stepping away from the Merge is the correct decision. Albie was right: Mum doesn't want this. Dad wouldn't have wanted us to merge either. He'd have been one of the thousands of people currently gathered outside the Clinic, shouting himself hoarse, demanding these experiments don't go ahead. My wanting this was selfish. I see that now.

All the ribbons are in place by the time Mum finally returns. Her dress, also Combine green, is high-necked with long, fluted sleeves, finished with delicate lace. Another gift from Nathan.

'Where've you been?' I ask, my voice sharper than I intended. 'We're supposed to be in Room One in a few minutes.'

'I had to talk to Nathan about something important,' she says. 'It won't take me long to get ready.' She's far calmer than I am, smiling at her reflection as I secure the ribbons in place. 'Mary and I always played with each other's hair when we were girls,' she says. 'We'd take it in turns. I often closed my eyes as she plaited or brushed. The feel of her hands would almost send me off to sleep. You were never keen on having your hair touched. You'd moan when I tried to style it for school. It's a shame. Your father and I always thought French plaits would suit you.'

'There,' I say, stepping back. 'What do you think? I've kept the ribbons to the minimum. It looks better that way. You've got these two here, in the front, and then one more at the back.'

'They're so lovely,' she says, her smile genuine. 'We should wear them more often.'

Nathan accompanies us to Room One.

'It's perfectly normal to feel apprehensive before your Ceremony,' he says as we walk down the corridor. 'In fact, it's a good sign – it means you're truly thinking about your decision. The weight of it. It shows you care. It wouldn't be natural to be Committing without any nerves. Everyone has moments of doubt.'

'We're not doing it, Nathan,' I say. 'We've made up our minds.'

'About what?' Mum whispers.

I shake my head, eyes wide, warning her to be quiet. She's been remembering the plan, then forgetting it, all morning. The last thing we need is Nathan thinking Mum still wants to go through with this, that I'm the one stopping her.

Annie, Ben, Noah and Lucas are already in Room One, standing together where the chairs are usually laid out. They stare at us in unison, as though they've already merged.

Mum smiles. She's the only one. Not even Lucas or Noah look happy. My stomach contracts. They know. They've already been told we're not joining them on the other side.

'Is everything okay?' I ask quietly.

Lucas nods, clearing his throat. 'It's the waiting,' he says. 'It's the worst part.'

Ben breaks away from the group. He begins pacing the room, biting his lip as he walks.

Nathan joins Callie and Angela by the door, where they talk in hushed voices. I catch Lara's name.

'Where are Jay and Lara?' I ask.

Nathan looks at me, his expression stern. 'They'll be here shortly,' he says.

Minutes pass. Still, no one other than the Support Workers has spoken.

Angela is now walking beside Ben, stroking his arm. 'Remember, you're fully prepared,' she says softly. 'You've spent the past three months getting ready for this moment. You're going to be fine.'

I look at the door, willing Jay and Lara to walk through it. We're running out of time. Mum stands with Annie, her eyes on the bump just visible beneath the robe. I think of our conversation in the nursery. *What if the baby doesn't make it?*

There's no time. I have to tell them now, say goodbye, even without Lara and Jay in the room.

'Mum and I need to tell you all something.' My voice cuts through the silence, unnaturally loud. Everyone turns to face me. 'We've… We've been talking about what this experiment actually entails, and about what could go wrong… We've decided to—'

The door swings open.

Jay enters, his arm round Lara's waist. She's pale and unsteady, leaning heavily against him as though his support is the only thing keeping her upright. Eliza follows them into the room.

'I left Lara to get ready for the Ceremony, and when I came back…' Jay's voice trembles as he clutches his daughter. Lara's head rests on his shoulder, her eyes closed, her mouth slack with saliva. Jay wipes his eyes with the back of his hand. 'She's taken something… Look at her. What's happening?'

Eliza places her hand on Jay's shoulder. 'We've had her thoroughly examined, Jay. Lara's going to be fine. The pressure of Committing today has taken its toll, that's all. She just needs to ride this out.'

Mum is already at Lara's side, wiping her chin as Jay fights back tears.

I step closer. 'You're not the only ones who won't be Committing,' I say, hoping to offer comfort. 'Mum and I aren't going to be in the Ceremony either.'

'We're still Committing,' Jay says, his voice firm. 'Kath and the boys need the Ceremony. They need the closure.'

Lucas frowns at me. 'You're not Committing? But you're still merging, right?'

Nathan steps in before I can answer. 'Laurie and Amelia are experiencing pre-Ceremony nerves,' he says. 'It's incredibly common and nothing to worry about.'

I shake my head. 'We've been weighing up the risks. It's too much of a gamble. If this is what you want, we still support you, but we can't—'

'Oh my god,' Ben says. 'This is what I was telling Annie last night. This has never been done before. We don't know that it's going to work. What if it goes wrong? What if we... what if we lose our baby?'

'Enough,' Eliza says. 'Let's bring the temperature down, shall we? Amelia, Laurie, this is entirely your decision. You have every right to back out. No one is going to stop you. But I implore you, don't push your own anxieties onto your friends.' She checks her watch. 'There will be time after the Ceremony to sit with your Partner and make your final decision. For now, everyone in The Oasis is waiting to celebrate you. Get through the Ceremony, and then decide.

'This is a celebration, remember. A coming together of your most trusted and loved ones. They're here to pay their respects to your bravery, your selflessness, your union. The Circle of Support is complete, and your guests are ready. Put your concerns aside for now. Bask in the love of those who cherish you, those who truly support your sacrifice. Enjoy this moment together. Enjoy the touch of your Partner and know that, in the days ahead, the two of you will become closer than ever before.'

She smiles. 'Annie and Ben, you're up first.'

Neither of them move. Their eyes are fixed on Lara, who is still slumped against Jay, her eyes closed, her mouth slack and lolling open. Mum gently pats her cheek, imploring her to stay awake, to stay with us.

'She's going to be okay,' Eliza says firmly. 'Come on now, you two. Don't disappoint your guests.'

Amelia

The Oasis looks truly beautiful. Every wall, save for the polished glass panels overlooking the Thames, is covered with flowers in full bloom. Fairy lights drape along the ceiling, glowing warmly between the floral chandeliers. Long tables, covered in white cloth, line the perimeter of the room, holding floral arrangements and candles.

Nathan has been surprisingly accommodating. After a quick chat with Eliza, he accepted our decision to back out and allowed us to be Witnesses, assigning us stools in the innermost ring. 'There will be time after the Ceremony to say your goodbyes,' he said. 'Just be mindful about the nature of your farewells.'

We stand with Kath and her sons, Annie's parents, Ben's brothers, Lucas and Noah's parents, and Ellie, our arms linked round each other's shoulders. Lara and Jay, the final pair, make their way slowly down the aisle. Lara shuffles clumsily, leaning heavily on her dad. Beside me, Kath lets out a shaky breath.

When Lara and Jay reach the centre, the Circle of Support closes around them. The Officiant bows their head, and we follow suit.

I glance upwards. Lara's eyes are now open, but they look distant, her mouth closed tight. Jay cradles her to keep her from falling. Unease coils in my stomach. The longer I watch, the more I feel the urge to intervene. I open my mouth to speak, then close it.

The Officiant raises their arms. 'Our beloved Participants are about to embark on a journey that will unite them in one body. They will merge, not only through their bodies, but through their souls, their minds, and their hearts. Let us thank all souls for their sacrifice: Benjamin Joseph, sacrificing his body; Annie Elizabeth, sacrificing her independence; their unborn child, sacrificing their nuclear family unit. Lucas Isaac, sacrificing his health; Noah Edward, sacrificing his body; their parents, sacrificing their sons. Jay Richard, sacrificing his sobriety; Lara Catherine, sacrificing her autonomy; their family, sacrificing their dear husband, daughter and sister.'

'We thank you for your sacrifice,' the Circle intones, heads still bowed.

All I can focus on is Lara, standing there, barely present. She's not sacrificing her autonomy; it's being stripped away. The urge to speak up builds again, but my throat tightens. Who am I to speak when her own mother stands here silent beside me?

I swallow hard, lowering my gaze.

'I ask you, our beloved Participants, to raise your heads and look now at the Circle, those bowing their heads in respect and admiration of your sacrifice. Let the bodies surrounding you bring you peace as we say together the Promise of the Witnesses.'

Together, the Circle speaks. 'We, the Witnesses of your blessed and selfless union, vow to support and love you forever more. We vow to be an ally, for you and all Combines who have made the sacrifice for the good of the many. We vow to love you now, then and always.'

The Officiant smiles. 'Please be seated.'

We sit. Annie and Lucas kneel on the embroidered cushions in front of Ben and Noah. But Jay doesn't move. He can't let go of Lara, whose eyes are now tightly closed, her body limp in his arms.

'I find the Thanksgiving to be the most special part of the Ceremony,' the Officiant says. 'It is so easy to go about our lives without stopping to reflect and to give thanks. Taking the time to do so, to express gratitude, is a meaningful practice. Witnesses, the responses are listed in your Order of Service.'

Ben begins. He takes a breath before lowering his chin to his chest. 'I thank my body for the good health I have been so fortunate to experience.'

The Circle responds in unison. 'We thank the physical body of Benjamin Joseph.'

Annie looks up at her fiancé. She reaches for his hand. 'I thank Benjamin Joseph's body for dancing with me, for walking with me, for pleasuring me and sleeping beside me. I thank Benjamin Joseph's body for the sacrifice it will endure to ensure our child has a future.'

'We thank the physical body of Benjamin Joseph.'

Noah goes next. His voice is quiet, as though he's speaking more to himself than to us. 'I thank my body for its resilience and strength, for enduring my illness long enough to allow me to be here, to do this.'

'We thank the physical body of Noah Edward.'

Lucas tucks his chin to his chest, as though in prayer. 'I thank Noah Edward's body for providing so many years of fun and mischief. I thank his body for healing, time and time again, and waiting for this miracle before giving up. I thank his body for everything.'

'We thank the physical body of Noah Edward.'

Lara remains silent, supported like a corpse in her father's arms. I wait for the Officiant to notice, to intervene, to stop the Ceremony. But nothing happens. They skip over Lara and smile at Jay. He clears his throat, his voice quavering. 'I thank the body of Lara Catherine for providing our family with so much joy. I thank the body of Lara Catherine for those years of bliss, for making our lives richer.'

'We thank the physical body of Lara Catherine.'

All eyes are on Lara. Kath covers her face with her hands, unable to watch. Lara's eyes, though open, are vacant, glazed over as if she's barely conscious. The Support Workers stand stiffly, their eyes averted, as though they, too, can't bear to watch.

The Officiant raises their arms again. 'Benjamin, Noah and Lara, your bodies will be sacrificed for the good of the world. Your unity is one of love, of selflessness and respect. My dear Participants, do you vow to always love and cherish one another, to support each other through every challenge that comes your way and to celebrate each other's triumphs?'

The answer comes as one, steady and rehearsed.

'We do.'

Lara's lips don't move. She stares ahead, empty.

'Do you vow to communicate openly and honestly with each other, to always listen to one another, and to never judge the other's thoughts and feelings?'

'We do.'

The Ceremony concludes, and we stand, our hands over our hearts, our heads lowered. 'We thank you for your sacrifice.'

We keep our heads bowed as our friends begin to leave the room. I lift my eyes just enough to see Annie and Ben walking out hand in hand, their faces pale. Lucas and Noah follow, smiling. As they disappear through the door, a thud breaks the silence.

Lara has slipped from her dad's grip and collapsed on the floor.

Kath cries out.

Eliza hurries over as Jay quickly scoops Lara up and carries her limp body out of the room. The doors close behind them, leaving the Witnesses standing in uneasy silence, our hands still pressed to our hearts. I scan the room for a videographer, someone documenting the Ceremony, gathering the evidence I need. But there isn't one. No cameras at all.

The Officiant raises their arms. 'Two hearts, one soul. Joined in spirit and bound by love. As we move to celebrate the merging of our beloved Participants, let us remember Our Combine, and the gift that they have bestowed upon the world.'

'From what was,' we chorus, 'Combines emerge anew. Their past we honour, their future we embrace. In the Merge, we protect their place.'

The Witnesses begin to file out silently. The outer ring leave first, uncoiling like a slow, deliberate serpent as they walk single file along the aisle of petals. The middle ring follows, their steps measured, steady. Finally, our ring joins the procession, with Mum and me at the back of the line.

As we reach the archway, hands seize my arms, yanking them roughly behind me. Panic surges. I open my mouth to scream, but a hand clamps over it. I struggle, twist, my eyes darting frantically to Mum.

She's been grabbed too, her cries stifled by another hand.

PART TWO

The Village

There's a light high above us, a bluish sun, illuminating but not heating the room. A man comes to our bedside. The blue intensifies as he leans over us, blotting out the sun. We close our eyes. The darkness has so many colours. It blooms and collapses like a jellyfish. The jellyfish we saw in the sea off Lyme Regis. A tiny city beneath the waves.

'Hello, Laurie-Amelia,' the man says softly. 'Don't be shy. Look at me.'

We don't want to look at him, but our eyes open and his are less than six inches away. Our vision is hazy. It takes a while for his face to come into focus. His eyes are deep brown, almost black, so dark that it's difficult to separate the pupil from the iris. It's the surgeon. He's younger than we remember, although we saw him only a few hours ago. Perhaps that's because we're older now – collectively – than we were before.

'That's better,' he says. 'How are you feeling?'

We say nothing.

'I'll give you something to drink in a moment,' he says. 'It tastes horrible – sorry – but it'll help stabilise you.' He produces a bright-red pencil from his top pocket and prods our right cheek with the blunt end. 'Can you feel that? Nod if you can feel it.'

We nod. It takes some effort; our head is too heavy for our neck.

He does the same with the other cheek. 'Can you feel that? Is the sensation comparable? Is it sharper, maybe? Duller perhaps. Nod if it's the same.'

There's a woman standing beside the surgeon. She's tall, angular, her smile a thin slit in her face. 'Hello, Laurie-Amelia.' She gives us a small wave. Her joints look odd, her movements too stiff, like she's a marionette.

We look back at the blue light.

There's a spill of memory: the sun when we left the Clinic, casting such long shadows. Stilt people, we said, and we laughed. We laugh now, a real laugh that the surgeon and the puppet woman can hear. They exchange a look.

The surgeon pockets his pencil and puts his hand out flat. The marionette woman places a small silver torch in his palm. How long must they have been working together to communicate this way, to understand one another with only a glance?

'Look up,' the surgeon says.

We flinch. The torchlight is powerful, a concentrated heat on our iris. Sunlight focused through a magnifying glass. A leaf ready to catch fire.

You've never liked eyes. Even as a little girl. You couldn't bear to watch when I put my contact lenses in. It always made you squirm to see my fingertip so close to my eye.

We didn't feel our mouth move, our jaw loosen. There's a ripple of panic. We steady ourselves, gripping the slippery mattress. We don't need our vocal cords to communicate with each other anymore. We were told this. It's one of the benefits, Eliza said. It'll save so much time, she insisted, those not-wasted seconds mounting up relentlessly.

The surgeon clicks off the torch and passes it back to the puppet woman. We blink the room into focus as he takes our hand. 'Give me a good squeeze, Laurie-Amelia. As hard as you can.'

We squeeze.

The surgeon smiles, satisfied, and takes our other hand. 'Again,' he says. He waits, frowns. 'And again.'

A memory rises: the peach walls of our kitchen, the large

wooden clock that didn't work properly, perpetually running five minutes fast or slow. Never on time. Our hands interlocked as we pushed against one another, battling to reach opposite sides of the room. Our laughter making us weak.

That's right. You always claimed you were stronger than me. Now's your chance to prove it.

We squeeze.

'That's better.' The surgeon pulls his hand from ours. 'Now for that drink I promised.'

It's not so much a drink as a syringe of liquid fire that he injects between our lips. Our tongue is scorched, and we cough and splutter as the burn spreads into our throat and beyond. We wince, our eyes shut tight, as the woman holds us down. We begin to writhe, feeling her hard wooden hands pressing on our shoulders.

'I'm sorry, Laurie-Amelia,' she says. 'I know it's not pleasant, but you must keep still.'

Our body convulses, a shared, instinctive rebellion. The pain is unbearable, but beneath it there's something else. Something worse. A creeping realisation, sharp and suffocating. We inhale sharply.

'I know, I know,' she murmurs. 'It'll pass.'

But it's not the burning in our throat that causes the ache. Not the agony of the procedure.

It's the truth.

Neither of us wanted this.

The surgeon smiles sympathetically. 'It'll be a nasty few days,' he says. 'But you'll get there, Laurie-Amelia. We'll do what we can to make the experience as painless as possible.' He pulls up the sleeve of our gown. 'You may feel a slight scratch.' We scrunch our eyes tight again as he injects us. 'There we go,' he says, withdrawing the needle. 'You sleep now, Laurie-Amelia. Get some rest.'

The light wakes us. The bulbs in the sconces above the bed gradually brighten until they glow with enough strength to reveal the walls and ceiling. The chest of drawers. The large, frameless mirror opposite the bed, rectangular but for its gently curved edges. Beneath the bed, a shaggy rug covers the majority of the oak floor. A soft landing should we fall.

It's the same every morning; first comes the light, then the announcement.

The voice is gentle, ethereal, dreamlike. It slips into our sleep, guiding us from the darkest corners of our mind, pulling us from haunted dreams: private recollections, resurrected as we sleep. Most mornings we wake shaking, saturated in sweat. Our bedsheets and pyjamas require changing. When this happens, Nathan mops our brow with a cold, damp flannel to calm us. 'What happened?' he asks, dabbing at our clammy forehead. But we can never tell him. The moment we wake, the memories collapse into nothing, leaving only the feeling of panic and shame.

The announcements vary. Some mornings, we're woken with a message of gratitude for our sacrifice; other times it's a reminder of what the Combine community strive to overcome. This morning, it's an affirmation: we are a beacon of strength, a catalyst for positive change, an indispensable force shaping the destiny of our rejuvenated world. We do as the voice instructs, repeating the affirmations as we stare at the faint spiral pattern etched into the ceiling. The pattern is so delicate it's often invisible.

A secret, intended just for us.

We lift our arm and point, our finger tracing the spiral pattern in mid-air. 'I am a beacon of strength,' we say, our arm sketching large circles. 'I am a catalyst for positive change.' Our movement slows, our tracing becomes more precise. 'I am an indispensable force shaping the destiny of our rejuvenated world.'

We've lost count of how many mornings it's been, how often this voice has woken us, how many of our days have begun with the almost imperceptible brightening of the room.

This morning, the sheet beneath us is dry. We shift over, lift the duvet, and run our palm over the sheet just to make sure. Yes. Bone dry. That makes it three mornings in a row. Nathan will be pleased. Proud. 'You're making such progress, Laurie-Amelia,' he'll say.

We've woken feeling calmer than usual. Whatever haunted our subconscious was only frightening enough to dampen our pyjama top. It clings to our stomach and sticks to our ribs. Dark patches have formed beneath what remains of our breasts.

We're so thin. Too thin.

We push ourselves up to a sitting position and consider our reflection in the mirror. Our hair hangs limply, reaching our navel, badly in need of a cut. Our cheeks and jaw are prominent beneath our pale skin. It's been so long since we've been outside, since we've felt the sun. We wonder if the sun is shining now, or if it's still dark out. The bedroom has no window. It makes it easier in a way. Waking to a blue sky, knowing we couldn't go outside, would be unbearable.

We can see the outside from the lounge should we want to. It still feels like a luxury. For a long time, we were confined to this room. We knew nothing of the outside, not the weather, not if it was light or dark, hot or cold.

We knew only this room, this mirror.

Everything in the apartment is muted: the walls are painted nutmeg, the tables and chairs made from plain blond wood; the carpet is cream. 'The soft tones allow you to acclimatise more easily,' Nathan explained when we questioned the bland decor. 'It would be a nuisance to have to wear your sunglasses all the time, wouldn't it?'

It's bright colours we find difficult. Reds, oranges and pinks are the most challenging, their vibrancy causing our eyes to water and our head to pound. Some days, even the plum colour of Nathan's tunic has us reaching for our sunglasses.

He sits beside us on the oatmeal-coloured sofa, his feet resting on the matching footstool. His shoes are still on, dirtying the fabric. He's looking out of the windows. They're floor-to-ceiling, offering a panoramic view of the complex. There's the occasional pulse of brightness from the overcast sky as it struggles to block out the sun. 'How are you feeling today, Laurie-Amelia?'

We try to respond to Nathan, but our mouth remains shut. *Please don't, Amelia. Please don't respond on my behalf. I can't stand you speaking for me.*

Speak to him yourself, then. Tell him how you feel.

Our mouth opens, but no sound follows.

I can't. I don't know how.

'I saw Noah-Lucas and Lara-Jay this morning,' Nathan says, lowering his feet and leaving scuff marks on the footstool. We'll scrub them clean later if we have the energy. 'They're both doing really well. We walked around the grounds. Right up to the lake and back. It was beautiful. So cold the grass crunched underfoot. Even the cobwebs were covered in frost.'

We consider the dirt, the imprint of their travels. Regret rumbles through us. How we wish we'd been on that walk, or even caught a glimpse of it. We lose hours staring out of the windows, observing the goings-on in The Village, searching for someone we know. We've never managed it. We watch unfamiliar Combines, trying to decipher what's different about them. Why they've been allowed out.

As nice as the apartment is, with its spacious rooms and high ceilings, it still feels confining. Suffocating. We yearn for fresh air, for the simple joy of wandering outside, feeling the earth beneath our feet. We daydream about being barefoot, feeling dew-kissed grass between our toes, the gentle sun warming our face.

The head-talk is all that keeps us sane. If we didn't have each other to talk to, the silence, the seclusion, would be insufferable.

'Noah-Lucas is desperate to see you,' Nathan continues. 'They're dying to know you're okay. I tell them you're doing well, but they're reluctant to believe me.'

I don't blame them. We must be the only ones they haven't seen.

We try to voice this thought but, again, no words form. We sigh loudly and rest our head against the sofa cushion. *Go on then. Speak for me.*

'Are we the only one from our group who hasn't been outside yet?'

Nathan considers our question. He's careful with the information he shares. For whatever reason, he's reluctant to speak about the others. He'll mention when he's seen them, tell us they're doing well and asking after us, but never much more. 'I don't want you comparing yourself to them,' is his usual explanation when we become cross about how little he divulges.

He must feel we deserve a treat today, as he shakes his head. 'Benjamin-Annie is still confined to their residence,' he says. 'They're doing really well, though, just as you are. I'm sure they'll be out and about soon.'

We've had a taste. We want more.

'Does Benjamin-Annie also see things that aren't there?' we ask. 'What happened earlier with the walls, does that happen to them, too?'

When Nathan arrived this morning, he found us crouching in the corner of the bedroom, our head tucked between our legs. 'The walls are moving in again,' we said, our voice shaking. 'Get on the floor or they'll crush you.'

Nathan joined us in the corner, rubbing our back as we rocked. 'The walls aren't moving, Laurie-Amelia. It's your brain playing tricks on you again. It will pass. It always does.'

We lifted our head to see if he was right. He wasn't. We quickly tucked our head back in, holding tightly to our knees, shaking as we waited for the walls to crush us.

'Don't you remember the night you were convinced there were shooting stars above your bed?' Nathan's palm moved in small circles on our back. 'Or the time you thought it was raining upwards? You said you could see puddles in the sky.'

Now, he looks away from the windows and turns to us. He doesn't smile our question away, doesn't brush it off as he usually does. 'I'm certain Benjamin-Annie will be experiencing hallucinations just as you are,' he says. 'A newly combined brain has to come to terms with a bombardment of thoughts and memories. A barrage of information. It's a major adjustment. Hallucinations are to be expected. If you think back to your time in the infirmary, when you were plagued with visions almost constantly, it's clear to see how far you've come.'

We close our eyes, trying to recall the days we spent in the infirmary. We see glimpses: the endless stream of doctors and nurses, the needles, the IV drips, the pain relief – but no hallucinations. No vivid images, no solid memories of what came before, or next. 'It's so difficult to remember,' we murmur. 'Everything is muddled and patchy.'

'Don't worry about the blanks, Laurie-Amelia. The memories will return to you eventually.'

His words provide no comfort. No matter how hard we try or how intensely we focus, the day of, and the days surrounding, our Merge remain a blur of confusion. We remember no lead-up to the Ceremony, no final sessions, no goodbyes with Albie or Mary. In fact, we recall no farewells at all. No Ceremony. Only a vague sense of anticipation and uncertainty, with occasional flashes of deep-purple fabric and the distant strains of the Ceremony March.

We haven't dared to voice what we fear might be true: that these fragments of memory are nothing more than our imagination, born from Nathan's countless retellings of that day. Our final day.

'How long were we in the infirmary?' we ask, our eyes still tightly shut.

'Seventeen days,' Nathan says. 'Though I'm sure it feels longer to you. My last Combine spent almost a month in the infirmary, and they told me it felt considerably longer. You coped incredibly well, Laurie-Amelia. Some Combines take up to two months to stabilise.'

We force ourselves back there, to the place we've spent so much time remembering. Not the beginning, but as far back as we can go – to our first memory. As uncomfortable as it is to think about, we must.

Was it day, or night? We're still unsure. It was impossible to keep track of time, to distinguish one from the other; our waking hours were a disorientating mixture of pain and fatigue. The infirmary was twilit and sinister viewed through our dark lenses. Medical posters lined the walls. *Merging Stages*, *Pain Management Techniques*, *Nutrition for Recovery*. One poster explained breathing exercises, showing a photograph of a man assailed by red arrows indicating the direction of his airflow. We tried to memorise the instructions but were never able to put what we remembered into practice. In the height of our pain, even something as simple as breathing seemed impossible.

We feel Nathan's hand on ours. 'Don't put so much pressure on yourself to remember. Think of the positives. You coped so well with this morning's hallucination. It only took you twenty minutes to recover this time. That's real progress.' He smiles. 'Now, I'm keen to see this demonstration of the intrusive memories that you promised me. I brought along the art supplies you requested. I've set them out on the table for you.'

We follow Nathan through to the dining room. We sit at the oval-shaped table, large enough for eight. Above us, a chandelier of tiny opal glass shades hangs like a cluster of stars, evoking old Hollywood. Often, when we eat, we imagine we're starlets beneath the chandelier's glow, being captured in black and white, later to be projected on screens across the world.

We gesture towards the paints, paintbrushes, palette and paper laid out in front of us. 'Just try something simple,' we suggest. 'The sky, or the ocean.'

Nathan looks at us with an amused expression. 'I'm painting?'

We nod.

He chuckles as he squirts some cerulean blue onto the palette and picks up the brush. 'Don't judge me. I'm no artist.' As he goes to dip the brush in the paint, we add a dollop of chrome yellow on top, covering the blue.

Nathan stares at the yellow. 'It completely takes over?'

We nod, take the paintbrush from him and begin swirling the yellow into the blue. 'You have to force the memory away to let other things come through. But often the memories don't improve, they just shift. Sometimes they get worse. If you're lucky, though, the memory becomes something safe, something you recognise. It's not blue anymore or yellow, but green. And green is familiar.'

We brush the paper with green. The motion feels strange, both instinctive and hesitant. Our strokes are heavier than we're used to, lacking the precision we once relied on.

We pass the paintbrush back. 'Why don't you finish off?'

Nathan takes the brush, ready to begin, but before he can, we reach out, grab a shock of cadmium red and streak it boldly across the green. The red cuts through, sharp and vivid, obliterating the green in places, distorting it in others.

Nathan pauses, his eyes following the red as it overtakes the canvas. 'It'll get easier to cope with,' he says quietly. 'The memories won't feel so consuming forever. They'll stop intruding like this. It just takes time.' He looks at us. 'When does it happen? Is there a pattern to it? A time of day, perhaps?'

We shake our head. Some memories come slowly, gradually shifting into focus like photographs developing in a darkroom. We enjoy watching them form. It's the traumatic memories that we don't want to share, or experience, that are intrusive. They come without warning, blinding us, making it impossible to see anything else. There's no predicting when the most problematic memories will surface, bringing with them pain and disgust. No way to know when our secrets, regrets and fantasies will burst forth, forcing us to witness the unveiling of our most private selves.

The worst are the sexual memories. These recollections are unbearably explicit. We see Albie, feel him, his warm moist mouth on our neck, his kisses scampering over our stomach, along our hips and between our thighs. Our body betrays us, becoming aroused despite our repulsion and suffocating embarrassment.

We try to force the memories away, but so often they resolve into something worse. It's no longer Albie we're with, but Mitchell. When this happens, we panic, scream and flail, demanding sedation. Nathan tries to calm us, encouraging us to use the techniques he's drilled into us, ways to look past the memories.

We never manage it. Each time, we're left to endure it, powerless to escape. Afterwards, it feels as though something inside us has been violated. We're left with a lingering sense of shame. We feel tainted. Unclean.

Nathan sighs, his eyes back on the blood-drenched canvas. 'I'll see what I can do to help, Laurie-Amelia. Maybe we can alter your medication, see if that makes a difference.'

We close our eyes and wonder, again, how we got here.

We're in the back of the old Ford Anglia. Our mother sits in the passenger seat, singing loudly and out of tune to Buddy Holly. Tony's laughing as he drives. The window is open, and we reach out. Our fingers cut through the rush of air as the wind pulls at our small hand, wanting to play. Mother's opening a packet of wine gums. They shine like jewels. She reaches back and places three in our outstretched hand. We gaze at them: two rubies, one emerald.

Our fingers close tightly round the sweets, and we shove all three quickly into our mouth. Tony doesn't like us having sugar. It gets us all worked up, he says, turns us stupid. We see him in the rear-view mirror, his eyes fixed on the road, his mouth still curved into a smile. A car pulls out in front of us, and Tony hits the brakes. One of the sweets goes down, unchewed, lodging in our throat. We panic, try to cough, but we can't.

Our hands flutter towards our mother, but we can't reach her.

She's trying to calm Tony, who's swearing loudly about the *fucking idiot* in front. The sweet in our throat is restricting our breath. We fumble with the seatbelt, leaning forward to grasp our mother's shoulder. Finally, she turns.

Tony's pulling over. Mother's unbuckling her seatbelt and scrambling into the back seat. She delivers a series of quick, desperate blows to our back, each one more urgent than the last. The sweet dislodges.

Finally, we can breathe again.

Then we're home, and she's telling us to stay in the car, not to come inside. She'll be right back, she says. It won't be long. We nod, eyes stinging, as Tony takes her hand and pulls her towards the house. We do as we're told, sitting quietly in the car, watching the front door.

When she emerges, her eye is swollen, and her nose is bleeding.

We jolt awake, our heart racing. The room is fully lit, and the announcement is in progress. *Stronger than the non-Combines, in more ways than one. You have earned the right...*

We sit up, the damp sheet clinging to us like a second skin, the duvet clenched tightly in our hands. Our breath comes fast, shallow, as we fight to steady it, trying to hold on to the fading edges of the dream, hoping it might fill in the blanks, reveal something about our final days before the Merge, or offer a hint of how we ended up here.

I remember a car. At least, I think it was a car. It might have been a train. And coughing. Were you coughing, or was I? Do you remember anything, Mum? We should write it down.

I don't. Not a thing. I'm sorry, Amelia. I'm useless.

Nathan arrives and coaxes us out of bed. He gives us our medicine. 'Go and shower,' he says quietly, his fingers already working the buttons on the duvet cover. Now that we're up, he won't look at us; his eyes are fixed on the soiled bedding beneath his hands. He gets cross when we wet the bed, like we've done it on purpose – like we meant to make things harder for him.

We head to the bathroom. As we undress, we try to piece together the gaping holes in our memory, the week-long voids that demand answers. But it's as futile as ever. There's nothing. No whisper of clarity. Only the truth – that we never wanted this. We both feel it, the unease, the regret. But it pulses stronger from Laurie than Amelia, a sharper pain, more insistent. What we can't recall, what stays frustratingly out of reach, is whether we ever voiced these doubts to each other. Did we know, back then, that both of us were sceptical? Or is this realisation something we've only come to understand now that it's too late?

Nathan doesn't like us to dwell on it. 'You mustn't fixate,' he says whenever we bring it up. 'It's unhealthy to obsess over something with no answer.'

We go round in circles, turning the question over and over in our mind. Did we avoid confronting our fears back then? Or did we bury them so deep that we tricked ourselves into believing we were ready? No matter how many times we go through it, we always arrive at the same conclusion: we couldn't have confronted each other. We couldn't have spoken openly about our doubts because, if we had, we never would have gone through with it.

The thought of our silence, of keeping so much from each other, makes us so unbearably angry. A relentless cycle of blame runs through our mind almost constantly: *If only you'd spoken up. If only you'd been honest with me.*

We've asked Nathan about the day we Committed more times than we can count, trying desperately to understand. 'Did we seem nervous?' we ask, each time hoping for a different answer.

'You had doubts, yes,' he always replies. 'But so many Partners do. It wasn't anything unusual. You were second-guessing yourselves, but deep down you knew you wanted to go ahead with it. Don't you remember us talking about this just yesterday, Laurie-Amelia?'

Though we do our best to resist him, Albie joins us in the shower. His wet body presses against ours as he wraps his arms round our waist, his hands on our breasts. We turn the water to the coldest setting. But the shock doesn't disrupt the hallucination. *Don't let this happen again. Block it. Please, Amelia.* We try to focus on the rapid cooling of our body: the goosebumps forming on our skin, our muscles contracting, our breath catching in our chest.

None of it works.

We turn, and Albie's fucking us. One hand grips our waist, the other tightens round our throat. 'Fuck, I've missed you.' His lips brush our earlobes, his warm breath tickling our ear as his hands move to our hips. We can't resist him. We lean back, giving in to our desire.

But then it's not him. Not his hand. Not his voice. We shake our head, forcing him off before he can fully contort into Mitchell. We shut off the water and step, dripping, from the shower.

We stand, shivering, pushing the memory away. We try not to argue, but it's impossible. No thoughts are private anymore. No matter how hard we try.

I didn't do it on purpose, Amelia. You think I want you experiencing my sex life? For god's sake. I've no more control over these things than you have. How do you think it makes me feel when you think of Albie like that? Everything you're imagining he's doing to you, he does to me. It's vile. He's like a son to me.

Like a son. Not your actual son. That's the difference, Mum. Dad is my actual dad. And you always contort it. Always take over.

I don't mean to. And I don't appreciate what you're implying. It's no worse for you. Being choked by Albie like I'm some sort of—

Fucking hell, Mum. Don't. Just forget it. Please.

It's not that easy.

Why? You manage to forget everything else.

As we dry ourselves, we continue to argue. It's the same argument we have every time we want to forget, and the intensity of it brings on a headache. A dull throbbing behind the ears.

You blame me for the gaps. I know you do. You can't keep denying it, Amelia. It doesn't help anything. And I agree with you. It's happened. I know it has. Every forgetful moment, every lost thought. It's dementia. I've plagued you. I've condemned you to a life of suffering all because I was too weak to say no.

Nathan has filled the washing machine with our bedding. We can hear its mechanical mumbling. He's putting on the clean sheet, smoothing out the creases and checking the corners. He glances at us, smiles. He's calmed down.

Once satisfied with the bed, he slips his hands into his pockets and rocks back on his heels. 'I've made you some porridge. It's in the kitchen on the hotplate. I thought you should have a proper breakfast this morning, something to keep you going for your assessment. I've got a good feeling about today.'

We don't share in his good feeling. It's been less than a week since our last test, since Dr Swanscombe was here, observing us, her dark eyebrows knitted together in a permanent frown. On three occasions, Nathan has believed us ready to venture beyond the apartment. Each time, Dr Swanscombe has subjected us to intensive testing. We've had our blood taken, our eyes examined, our tolerance to noise levels and temperature variations tested. We've endured medical health screenings and adaptability tests. Each time, the process has exhausted us. And, each time, we've failed.

'Hurry up and eat your porridge, Lor.'

We jump, our spoon clattering onto the table. Our mother is sitting opposite us, holding a bloody tea towel to her head. She's more silhouette than substance, featureless but unmistakably her. She's wearing a dressing gown, the collar stained red. We blink, and she vanishes.

We focus on the spoon, its smooth bright metal. The curve and contour of its design, the weight of it in our hands. This is real. This is our anchor. Concentrate hard enough, and we'll stay grounded.

But then she's back, sitting beside us, her features still impossible to make out. The lines of her face blur and shift. 'We don't want you being late for school,' she says, bending to collect shards of a smashed plate. 'Help me, Lor. Let's get this picked up before he notices. Before he gets angry.'

'Laurie-Amelia.' Nathan's voice cuts through, his grip firm on our arms, holding them to our sides. 'Breathe with me.'

We do as instructed, matching his deep breaths. Eventually, our mother melts away. What remains is the bowl, our bowl, shattered on the floor.

We're standing in the kitchen opposite Dr Swanscombe, who is peering intently at our charts. She's a tall woman, and the purple tunic makes her shoulders appear menacingly broad. 'Your bloods are good,' she says, her untamed eyebrows arching slightly, 'as is your mobility. You're considerably stronger than you were last week, and Nathan tells me your appetite has returned to normal.'

We nod. Eating has become easier. We try to be democratic about food, alternating between our favourites, but it's difficult to know what they are anymore. Working out our combined palate has required perseverance and patience. Many of our favourite flavours when we were separate, we now can't tolerate. The smell of fresh fish, for instance, or the bitterness of coffee.

'Your physio reports are especially pleasing.' Dr Swanscombe's large finger moves along the notes. Her nails are sensibly filed, rounded and neat. 'Your improvement is quite commendable.'

Again, we nod. We're steady on our feet now and have no trouble carrying things anymore. The first time Dr Swanscombe observed us, we dropped the water jug and drenched her trousers.

'Perhaps you could show me your progress so I can see for myself. How do you feel about walking without your stick, Laurie-Amelia? It might be best to try in the lounge. The carpet will cushion you should you fall.'

That seems counterintuitive. We'll take more care, pay closer attention, if we walk on a hard surface.

Tell her that, Mum. Go on. Try to speak.

We try, but no words form. We lick our lips and try again. Nothing.

Dr Swanscombe's eyebrows converge at the centre. 'I thought you said they were making progress with their speech, Nathan.'

'I never specified—'

She raises her large hand, silencing him. 'I wonder what would happen if you refused to voice those trickier thoughts, Laurie-Amelia, the ones you're struggling to articulate.'

Is she telling you to ignore me?

'I'm not suggesting you ignore the thoughts,' she says, as though she's heard. 'Just that you don't speak them aloud. You need a reason to force those words out. Right now, there's no need for that part of your brain to connect with your vocal cords. If you stop speaking for that part of yourself, those thoughts will have to find another way out.'

It's not as though I don't want to speak, or that I'm not trying hard enough. No matter how much effort I put in, the words never... solidify – never become anything more than thoughts. You refusing to talk for me will only frustrate us. It won't make me try any harder. It's impossible for me to try harder, Amelia. Tell her. Tell her we're trying our best.

'We're trying our best.'

'We?' Dr Swanscombe purses her lips. 'I don't want to hear you referring to yourself in the plural, Laurie-Amelia. You must embrace your singularity.' She taps her temple. 'If you're not bonded in here, how can you possibly be bonded' – she points at her mouth – 'in here?'

We nod. We know she's right, but it's so difficult. It feels inauthentic to pretend we're one combined being. We're not. Not yet, at least.

'Can we walk... Can I walk – in the kitchen?'

'Why the kitchen?'

'I'll take greater care if the surface is hard. I'll pay more attention if there's a bigger chance of hurting myself.'

Thank you, Amelia.

Dr Swanscombe assesses the precision of our foot placement as we walk slowly around the lounge. We walk heel to toe, our arms outstretched for balance, just as she instructed. 'Very good,' she says eventually. 'You're wonderfully coordinated, remarkably steady compared to the last time I observed you. You've clearly been putting in the hours, Laurie-Amelia.'

We nod. We have worked hard. Even when we've wanted nothing more than to stay tucked up in bed, we forced ourselves to attend the physio sessions. We haven't missed a single one. Whenever one of us has groaned about going, the other made sure we got there.

'Take a seat.' Dr. Swanscombe gestures to the sofa before settling herself on the footstool. She begins flicking through the documents in her folder, moistening her finger with her tongue every few pages. 'I must say, I'm pleasantly surprised by how much you've progressed this past week. Last time I visited, you insisted on wearing your sunglasses. Now look at you, not even a squint and the lights are on full. I always find it remarkable how suddenly Combines can take a positive turn.'

Nathan's nodding eagerly. 'I told you, Doctor. They've come on leaps and bounds. Only yesterday—'

'Here we are.' Dr. Swanscombe pulls a green plastic card

from a clear wallet. She rummages in her bag for a lanyard and slips the card into the attached transparent pocket before handing it to us. 'You must wear this at all times when you're outside your apartment. It grants you access to communal spaces and serves as your identification. On the back of your card, you'll find your apartment number and emergency contact information should you require it.'

'You mean... I've passed? I'm allowed out?'

'Congratulations, Laurie-Amelia.'

We stare at the photograph on the ID card. It's of us – of Amelia – wide-eyed and smiling. We have no memory of the picture being taken. The white background provides no clues, nothing to help us retrieve the memory. We're wearing a plain black t-shirt, one that stirs no recollections. 'When was this taken?'

Nathan quickly takes the lanyard from us and slips it round our neck. 'Just before your Merge, Laurie-Amelia. Congratulations. I knew you could do it.'

I have no voice. How can we be ready to venture outside when I can't speak?

'You're sure I'm ready? What about the part of me that can't speak?'

Dr Swanscombe begins gathering her belongings. 'Consider my suggestion about not voicing those other thoughts. I think it could prove an effective method to get your whole self conversing.'

Our watch beeps. So does Nathan's. Our medication reminder. Nathan silences his watch, and we do the same. Dr Swanscombe thanks us for our sacrifice, and we thank her for her faith in us. We see her to the door as Nathan prepares our pills. She nods stiffly before walking away.

A strange woman.

We watch her go.

We leave our hair wet, the way we like it when we sleep. We never enjoyed the feeling of wet hair before, never found a damp pillow comforting like we do now. We didn't used to overheat at night.

We get into bed and pull the duvet up over us, sitting with our back against the headboard. We remove our wedding and engagement rings and place them on the bedside table. We can't seem to get used to wearing the jewellery at night. It upsets us. We'd never have removed them before. *So long as you don't let me forget to put them back on in the morning. Mitch would be devastated if we lost them. I would be devastated. We mustn't lose them, Amelia.*

We'd like to remove our watch, too. The strap feels constricting when we're trying to sleep. Claustrophobic, even. But we must wear it. It records our sleep and gives us a score upon waking. We've never tracked our sleep before. Neither of us were particularly good sleepers, and knowing we'd had a bad night before a long day at work wasn't appealing. 'Every Combine requires a minimum of ten hours sleep a night,' Nathan told us when we complained about wearing the watch at night. 'Preferably more. Without enough sleep, your recovery will take significantly longer. Your brain must be fully recharged to align. It's why I insist you nap most days.'

The lanyard is on the bedside table beside the rings. We pick it up and stare at the photograph. *Who do you think took the picture? Nathan? Or a professional photographer?* We bring the photograph closer to our eyes, searching for a clue, a detail that might unlock the memory. We look so happy. But there it is again. That nagging, unshakable feeling that we didn't want this, that our being here is due to a terrible misunderstanding. We close our eyes, willing the memory to surface, a glimpse of that final day.

Nothing.

I can't bear it. I can't stand the fact that I'm erasing your memories. We must tell them. We must ask for help. There has to be a way of reversing this. My body isn't underground yet.

Our legs tingle. A faint, buzzing current fuelled by anxiety. The thought of my body – Mum's body – our body – lying cold and lifeless in storage, waiting for the burial it deserves. We shake our head, refusing to let the panic settle.

Nathan has told us repeatedly to stop catastrophising. 'The memories will return,' he always says. 'Everyone struggles at first, Laurie-Amelia. You've just got to keep trying, keep willing those moments to come back to you, and they will. You'll see.'

As though summoned, Nathan enters the room. He hands us our tablets and a glass of water. We've lost track of how often medicine is given to us. We've no idea how many pills we swallow each day. At first, we tried to count, but it proved impossible. There are so many pills that at times we feel we can't swallow any more. Like this morning, when a part of us rejected them. We blocked our throat and spat them out. Nathan closed his eyes, barely containing his frustration. 'You're only hurting yourself, Laurie-Amelia.' He used a tissue to pick up the partially dissolved tablets. 'Without medication, you'll find the merging process intolerable. Far worse than this heartburn you're complaining about, I can assure you.'

This time, we swallow the tablets easily. Nathan takes the empty glass from us, then turns off the light and switches on a white noise machine in the corner of the room. It's something that never used to soothe us, but now we find it essential to quieten our mind. When we're trying to drift off, our head-talk can become tense.

Nathan checks that our watch has sufficient battery life. He pats us on the shoulder like a proud father. 'Well done,

Laurie-Amelia,' he says. 'I knew you could do it. You get a good night's rest. We've an adventure waiting for us tomorrow.'

We're in the woods. Or is it a park? We're surrounded by trees and twisted branches. We're being chased. There's laughter. It's coming from us. Giggles erupting like bursts of confetti.

Are we playing tag? Or stuck-in-the-mud?

We sprint, our boots churning up splashes of water and mud that clings to our legs. A large hand extends towards us from the sky. We speed up, slipping on the wet ground.

Our laughter morphs, distorts, becomes a cry.

We continue to run but lose our footing. A sharp pain shoots up our leg. The trees twist and dissolve, and we're running, stumbling down the driveway towards our house, holding a small child.

The front door.

We reach it, but the hand is back, closer now. It grabs for us. We duck.

Our ankle throbs. The child screams. But we keep running. Muddy footprints mark our passage through the doorway and up the stairs. We reach the bedroom. Slam the door shut. We take a deep breath, daring ourselves to look at our ankle. We see bone.

We crumple, and so does the child. His lungs give out.

Below, beneath the floorboards, lies our mother.

Trapped.

'Mum?'

Then she's gone. Downstairs. With him.

There's the sound of flesh meeting flesh. Her cries.

Then it stops. All is calm. We float upwards.

We welcome you to another beautiful day of healing and growth.

Up, up, floating like a bubble.

Nurture your merged mind, body and spirit as you continue on your journey of transformation. Let us support one another, uplift one another and celebrate each small victory along the way.

We sit up, gasping for breath. *Who was that man chasing us?*

But the moment we ask, we forget.

We hadn't anticipated the tranquillity of the world beyond the apartment. Nathan advised us to wear our sunglasses for our first outing, and through our lenses the corridor has a gentle, golden hue. Arched windows stretch along the walls, interspersed with delicate brass sconces. Soft classical music drifts from hidden speakers.

We walk slowly, Nathan's elbow tightly gripped in our left hand, our walking stick in our right. The indents left by the walking stick create a pattern on the plush carpet. We pass our neighbours' apartments, each door adorned with cursive brass lettering displaying the inhabitant's name. The names curl beneath the apartment numbers like a smile: Lucy-Elizabeth lives at number 32, Annalisa-James at number 33, Gary-Eleanor at number 34. We pause to consider the others who willingly merged. The names smile back at us, content in their decision.

'Well done, Laurie-Amelia,' Nathan says, gently pulling us forward. 'Keep on going.'

Nathan reminds us of someone from our childhood. It's his height, we think, the sense of safety he provides. The recollection takes a moment to solidify. Then it comes, just like that, the outline of him, perfectly clear in our mind.

Walter Green was his name. He lived opposite in a small bungalow. He put me up whenever I wasn't able to go home. He never asked questions, at least not to me. He just let me sit with him, playing board games until it was time for bed. I got to be very good at draughts... Sometimes he took me to school the next morning. He called the police once. My mother hated him for doing that, but I never did. I liked knowing he was there, looking out for us.

Our stomach knots with unease. *I wish you'd told me about all of this sooner. I'm so sorry, Mum.*

We push the memory away before it's able to take hold. It's surprisingly easy, just as Nathan said it would be. 'Really, Laurie-Amelia,' he assured us, helping us into our coat, a long black duffel sent from Mary to keep us warm in the cold weather. 'You'll find your new surroundings more interesting – more stimulating – than the memories of the past, and they'll win out. You've become too accustomed to your apartment. It's no wonder the memories consume you in here. You've been holed up inside for too long.'

We didn't like to ask him exactly how long it's been. It's November, we know that much. But how far into November are we? How many weeks, or months, have we been trapped inside with only Nathan for company? *If only we could remember the journey from the infirmary to the apartment. Just a whiff of the weather would help. Were we stretchered, do you think? Or wheeled? I doubt we could have walked. Perhaps we were carried?*

At the end of the corridor, a large window offers a view of the garden lined with evergreen bushes. It's been snowing. Not a great amount, just enough to dust the grey stone path that winds through the garden and leads to the pond. We wonder if it contains koi, their marbled bodies colouring the water like living strokes of paint.

'There are over three hundred acres to explore,' Nathan says. 'Much of the grounds here are forested, which is a real treat. Some Villages, the more urban ones, have very little nature for Combines to enjoy. Now, Laurie-Amelia.' His eyes soften the way they do when he's trying to comfort us. 'Being reunited with your friends will no doubt cause you some upset and confusion. You'll have conflicting ideas of these people, differing recollections. My advice is that you don't let the memories overwhelm you when they come. Remember the grounding work we've been practising. When you find yourself thinking back, focus on something in the here and now. A smell, or a physical sensation. Today, for this walk, try to be entirely present.'

The elevator dings, announcing its arrival. Nathan turns, tugging gently at our arm, but we remain where we are, staring out at the garden, our heart suddenly on overdrive. We press our palm against the window. 'Albie,' we whisper. 'Why is he...' But then he vanishes. There's no one there. Albie isn't by the pond, isn't tossing bread to the fish. *A hallucination?* Our stomach knots again, tighter this time. Albie was no more there than our mother was at breakfast yesterday morning.

Nathan guides us away from the window. The imprint of our palm lingers. 'We'll take it nice and slow once we're outside. One step at a time. You let me know if you want to go home and we'll immediately turn back.' He steps inside the lift, holding the door open with his arm.

We step inside.

'Well done, Laurie-Amelia.'

We look in the mirror. Amelia stares back at us. We're wrapped in a duffel coat, our hair covered by a winter hat. We think of the mirrors from the Clinic. There were so many of them, lined up in rows. But they weren't mirrors. Not really. *They did look like mirrors, though. If I'm remembering correctly.* We frown, and our reflection frowns back. *Did I spend a lot of time in the mirror room?*

Yes. You practised every day.

That's right. I spent all those hours contemplating my reflection.

But it wasn't you in the mirror. Don't you remember?

I can't—

The elevator doors open. We move cautiously into the lobby, not trusting the marble floor beneath our walking stick.

The foyer is grand, the high walls adorned with silver trees whose trunks and branches ascend, merging into a canopy of silver leaves. The central chandelier is directly above us, its fat crystal droplets catching the light. Nathan places a finger on our chin and gently lowers our head so that we're looking at him.

'It's a lot to take in, Laurie-Amelia. My advice is that you don't examine anything too closely. Exist on the surface. Allow yourself to experience the wonders of The Village without becoming overwhelmed.' He keeps his finger resting on our chin. 'Noah-Lucas and Lara-Jay are waiting for you by the entrance. Don't look. Focus on me. Listen to what I have to say. I want you to close your eyes and think of Noah-Lucas as they were before. I want you to remember Noah *and* Lucas. Let all your memories come forward. Don't push them away because they're contradictory or unpleasant. Just allow them the space they need.'

We do as Nathan says, closing our eyes. A deluge of memories immediately follows: We're in The Oasis, having lunch. Lucas is sitting both on our left and our right. He's telling a joke, and we're laughing, but he's also talking about something deeply distressing, and we're sad. We're at Annie and Ben's apartment, chatting to him. He's standing beside us, and he's a few feet away, talking to someone else.

We grip on to Nathan.

'Take control,' Nathan says calmly. 'Let it happen. See both boys as they were. Accept your memories as truth. Allow them to coexist.'

We're sitting in the circle, writing in our notebook, and Noah is watching us. Our eyes are on the page of notes, but we're watching him, too. He's holding our hand, walking with us out of the room, and we're watching him go, holding on to someone else. He's crying, his eyes red and tiny. He's laughing, his head thrown back.

'Okay,' Nathan says. 'That's enough now. Try and block the memories, refuse to let them continue. Return here. What can you smell, Laurie-Amelia? What can you feel?'

We hold and release our breath until our mind settles. *I smell polished wood, do you? It's subtle, but it's there. Really focus, and you'll catch the scent.* When we eventually open our eyes, Nathan is smiling. 'Spectacularly done, Laurie-Amelia. You controlled that wonderfully. Now, I want you to do the same thing for Lara-Jay. I suspect this will be a more emotional experience for you due to the nature of your relationship, how close you became and how much they opened up to you. Let's start with Jay.'

We observe our friends from a distance. They're standing in a cluster by the entrance. Noah-Lucas wears a thick navy-blue parka with a fur-lined hood, while Lara-Jay is wrapped in a long black wool coat. Callie and Eliza are dressed just like Nathan, in smart, plum-coloured overcoats. How comforting it is to recognise them all, to have their names come to us without hesitation. *I'd never have managed this before. It's working, Amelia. You're restoring my memory.*

Noah-Lucas is smiling, talking animatedly. Callie and Eliza are fully engaged in whatever Noah-Lucas is saying. Lara-Jay, however, is not. They're staring at the wall, their eyes on the silver branches.

We scan the lobby, but there's no sign of Benjamin-Annie. *They're not out yet. Remember what Nathan told us. They're still in their apartment.*

Lara-Jay spots us.

Our stomach lurches, our eyes stinging with unexpected grief.

She's in there, Mum. Just like you're in me. She sees you, just like you see her.

Lara-Jay points at us, and the others turn, joy spreading across their faces. Noah-Lucas hurries over, breaking into a run. 'Oh my god,' they say, reaching for us. They hug us tightly, and we're momentarily blinded by the memories. Something must give away our discomfort as Noah-Lucas quickly pulls back. 'I'm so sorry,' they say, blinking beneath their fringe. 'I didn't mean to startle you. It's just I've missed you so much.'

We wipe our eyes, wanting to return the sentiment, to tell them of the hours we've spent searching for them through the windows. We want to ask how they're feeling, if they're as healthy as they look, if they're cancer-free. But we made a promise. Neither of us will speak. Not until we can do it together. Nathan knows this; we were clear about our silence once we were out of the apartment.

'Laurie-Amelia may find talking trickier than you do, Noah-Lucas,' he explains. 'I'm sure they'll find their voice soon, but they're predominantly here for the outdoor exercise, and to enjoy your company.'

Noah-Lucas nods and squeezes our hand. 'That's okay. No need to talk. Just being here is enough.' They smile, light in their eyes. 'I did it, Laurie-Amelia. It worked. I don't have cancer anymore.'

We wrap our arms round them. They laugh, and the sound of it brings on more tears. Over their shoulder, we see Lara-Jay still standing with Eliza and Callie, who seem to be encouraging them to approach us. We release Noah-Lucas, wiping our eyes on our sleeve. Lara-Jay watches, unsmiling. Their arm is no longer outstretched, no longer pointing in our direction, but hanging limply at their side.

We look at their blank face, their cold stare.

Noah-Lucas follows our gaze. 'Don't worry about Lara-Jay,' they say quietly. 'Their hostility isn't personal. They've got more conflict than most of us. They've got further to go before they can feel fully aligned. But they'll get there, isn't that right, Nathan?'

'It certainly is.'

Lara-Jay holds our gaze, and we theirs.

I thought Nathan said they were doing well. They don't look well, do they?

'Let's get going,' Nathan says. 'It's about time you got some fresh air, Laurie-Amelia.'

The Village is very different from how it appeared through the apartment windows. The paths that snake around the grounds are wide and inviting, not narrow and restricting as they seemed from above. The air is crisp, the sky blank, the sun hidden behind thick cloud. Snow crunches underfoot as we walk between lawns bordered with manicured shrubs. Nathan's arm is linked with ours, while our other hand grips the walking stick. *Hold on tight, Amelia. It wouldn't do to take a tumble out here.*

Cycle lanes run parallel to the pedestrian paths, and Combines and Support Workers cycle past, ringing their bells in greeting. Nathan nods and smiles. Noah-Lucas waves and wishes them a good day. There are sheltered rest areas with cushioned benches, where Combines and Support Workers sit, enjoying the scenery: expansive lawns of a lush, deep green, so different from the parched, brown lawns of the outside world; vibrant flowerbeds and meticulously trimmed hedges, some shaped into archways and towering hedgerows.

We can't help but smile as we walk; the sheer relief of being outside is overwhelming, all-consuming. If only we were steadier, more certain of our balance, we'd spread our arms wide and sprint across the lawn. *Do you remember when you were young, and we'd race through the park? Your little legs would pump furiously. You were always so determined to win.*

We tilt our face to the sky, savouring the clarity of that memory. We've done it. We've merged, and now we're here, with friends, recalling memories we would have lost before. We must hold on to this feeling, this sense of success, of freedom, and not let it fade, not let it dissolve like snow on the gravel paths, pricked with the delicate footprints of birds.

Noah-Lucas chats happily, unconcerned by our slow pace. They tell us about the friends they've made and the activities they've been up to. 'My neighbour, Justin-Ray, is being signed off next week,' they say. 'You'll have to make sure you meet them before they go. They're hoping to study International

Relations at Oxford. Being a Combine was a condition of their entry. Isn't that cool?'

Lara-Jay follows behind us, one arm in Callie's, the other in Eliza's. We wonder why they don't have a walker or at least a stick. *Perhaps they need more support.* We keep turning our head, offering a smile. Each time, the Support Workers smile back, but Lara-Jay remains distant, as though they haven't noticed us at all.

'There's a lot going on here,' Noah-Lucas continues, 'so many workshops and events to aid our progression. So long as you're completing your therapy and physio sessions, you're free to join in with whatever you like in your spare time. Well, I have to go to school for three hours each day, but you won't have to do that. It's quite fun, actually. The teachers here aren't strict like the ones at my old school. They want you to enjoy learning. Did you know there's a journaling workshop? I think you'd enjoy it, Laurie-Amelia. You were always writing in your diary.'

Gratitude swells in our chest. *They remembered me, Amelia. They remembered that I'm here.* Noah-Lucas points excitedly at a glass building to our left. It gleams in the muted light, its glass walls reflecting the snow-dusted lawns and surrounding trees. 'This is The Village theatre. Did you know they had a theatre here? I didn't.'

'The shows are spectacular, Laurie-Amelia,' Nathan says, squeezing our hand. 'There are performances on the last weekend of each month. You should consider getting involved in a production once you're settled in. Combines have reported that being part of the company is extremely beneficial for their social progression and mental well-being. There was a performance of *Les Misérables* last week.'

'I went,' Noah-Lucas says. 'Callie encouraged me to. She says it's important to expand my horizons, that I should be open to enjoying things I didn't used to.'

'What was the verdict?' Nathan asks. 'Did you enjoy it?'

Noah-Lucas shakes their head. 'I'm not a fan of musicals. Never will be. It was a cut-down production, but still too long... Ben would have loved it, though. Sorry. Benjamin-Annie, I mean.'

We reach for Noah-Lucas's arm and widen our eyes. *Tell us*, we try to say, *tell us more about Benjamin-Annie.* They smile, understanding immediately. 'Benjamin-Annie isn't out yet. I don't know any more than you do. What I want to know is how *you* are, Laurie-Amelia. I haven't been told a thing. How's your memory? Can you remember things you didn't used to? Has it worked?'

Even if we were speaking, we wouldn't know how to respond. Sometimes, yes, we recall things we couldn't before the Merge. Other times, our mind is as blank as it ever was. It's like reaching into a fog, grasping for something that should be there, but isn't. How we got here, for instance, remains a mystery.

We continue along the path, moving away from the theatre. Behind us, Lara-Jay coughs loudly, a harsh, hacking sound that rattles their chest. We turn to see they've stopped walking. Eliza is patting their back. *They don't seem at all well, do they? Why did Nathan tell us they were doing well? And why doesn't Noah-Lucas seem concerned? I can't understand it.*

'Keep walking, Laurie-Amelia,' Nathan says. 'Don't make them feel self-conscious.'

Ask after them, Amelia. Go on, I don't mind you speaking. I want to know. We nod encouragingly. *Honestly, Amelia. Ask for me. I won't be upset. Make sure Lara's okay.*

We hold off asking for now, knowing we might change our mind. This tends to happen. Internally, we make an agreement, but then a part of us forgets we ever offered permission, and we argue terribly.

The path we're walking narrows. We pass a tall white-brick building that Noah-Lucas tells us is their apartment block. 'It's for sixteen- to eighteen-year-olds,' they say. 'It's fairly similar to yours, though, if your lobby is anything to go by. I think they just like to group Combines of similar ages together. It makes sense, I guess. I get on really well with most of the Combines in my block.'

'Yes,' Nathan says. 'The apartment blocks are allocated to optimise social interaction and promote a sense of community. Blocks are allocated according to the age of your Host body. So, in your case, Laurie-Amelia, everyone in your apartment block is physically twenty to twenty-five. That way, we're able to offer age-specific support tailored to the needs of residents.'

We consider what this means for us. No one in our support group was a similar age, so they won't be living in our block. But it would be simple enough to work out where Benjamin-Annie lives. All we'd have to do is observe, take notice of where the thirty-somethings are heading. We could stand outside their apartment and wave. We could visit them every day, give them what we so desperately craved: a friendly face.

'There are thirteen blocks,' Noah-Lucas continues. 'All the children up to the age of twelve live in a separate part of The Village. And the elderly Combines live in residential bungalows at the other end. That's right, isn't it, Nathan?'

'It is indeed.'

The path winds between an expanse of grass. To our right, a Combine sits at a bench, sipping from a thermos. A Support Worker, dressed in a plum-coloured overcoat, sits with them, chatting happily. They wave, and Noah-Lucas waves back. 'Do you have crazy dreams now?' they ask. 'I had this dream last night that I was a merman. I raced the dolphins. It felt so real.'

We remember this morning, our sheets damp with cold sweat.

We must cringe because Nathan pats our back reassuringly. 'Laurie-Amelia is suffering from night terrors,' he says. 'They can be rather – upsetting. But it's reassuring to know that Noah-Lucas is having good dreams, isn't it, Laurie-Amelia?'

Our nightmare last night caused us so much distress that we cried for the better part of an hour, more from embarrassment than anything else. It was so humiliating witnessing Nathan changing our soaking sheets, to have him privy to our terror.

It was Harrison we dreamed of. Losing him.

'That sounds horrible,' Noah-Lucas says. 'I had nightmares in the beginning. Don't worry, though. They don't last. The good dreams are incredible once you get there.'

We consider their earnest expression. It's difficult to imagine Noah-Lucas has struggled at all. They seem so incredibly well.

They nod. 'Honestly, I did. The nightmares were tough. I think mine must have been about cancer because I'd wake up believing that I was still ill. I *felt* ill. That's how convincing the dreams were. I had dreadful fatigue and aching bones. It felt just like it did before. I was convinced the fever and night sweats were a symptom of illness, rather than a reaction to the Merge. I quickly recovered, though. It didn't take long until I felt better.'

Nathan smiles. 'Noah-Lucas was out of their apartment in under fourteen days. Isn't that remarkable, Laurie-Amelia? It's rare you see a Combine coping so well so soon after their Merge.'

A group of runners, both Combines and Support Workers, jogs by in their workout gear, either Combine green or purple depending on their role. Each top features a golden mandala emblem. They smile and wave as they pass, their breath forming white clouds.

Nathan and Noah-Lucas stop walking. We wait for Lara-Jay to catch up. Each small step seems to demand immense focus. Without Eliza and Callie holding on tight, we imagine they might topple over. We're still in agreement about speaking, so we voice our concern. 'Is Lara-Jay really okay, Nathan? They seem so…'

Noah-Lucas beams, delighted by the sound of our voice. 'Spaced out?' they suggest.

'You have to consider their circumstances,' Nathan says, watching Lara-Jay's slow progression down the path. 'Jay and Lara were never close, even if they were a match. Their consciousness has further to come than yours does. Theirs is a much larger adjustment. They celebrated their Passing last week, so they're doing well, despite appearances. Like you, they're experiencing some difficulties with communication. You'll be a good person for them to have around, Laurie-Amelia. Their frustrations aren't too dissimilar to your own.'

They're like me? Trapped inside?

'A part of them can't speak?'

Nathan scratches his cheek. 'Neither part of them is able to speak. It's nothing to be concerned about,' he adds quickly. 'Like I said, everyone progresses at different rates. No two Combines are the same. Take Benjamin-Annie, for instance. They're not yet out of their residence, but they're doing very well. They're communicating wonderfully. It's their balance that's tricky. We're taking extra precautions due to their pregnancy. If they weren't pregnant, they'd no doubt be out in The Village, too.'

'They must be due soon.'

'They have just under a month to go,' Nathan says. 'It's extraordinarily exciting. We're incredibly lucky to be so involved in their journey.'

Eight months pregnant. I think that means the baby is the size of a pineapple. I always loved keeping track of how big you were when you were growing inside of me.

Lara-Jay finally catches up with us. 'Hi.' We smile. 'It's great to see you.'

It's Jay's body standing in front of us: the broad shoulders, the hat pulled low over his bald head. But there's something in the way they stoop, the slight downward turn of their mouth, that's unmistakably Lara.

'How lovely to hear your voice, Laurie-Amelia,' Callie says warmly. 'Good for you.'

'How are you feeling, Laurie-Amelia?' Eliza asks. 'The first outing can be an exhausting experience. Perhaps we should loop back? We could pass the art gallery. I can imagine you'll enjoy spending time there.'

'How are you, Lara-Jay?' we try again.

Nothing. Callie smiles, releases Lara-Jay's arm and comes to our side. She places a gentle hand on our back, guiding us forward. Nathan keeps hold of our arm. 'Don't worry about Lara-Jay,' she whispers. 'They're still processing everything. It took a while for Noah-Lucas to get used to them, too. They're fine. They've just got a lot going on inside their head.'

We pass a large red-brick Victorian-style building. 'The Margaret Hayes Art Gallery,' Callie explains. 'The Hayes family are one of our biggest donors. They've given millions to the Combine cause. There are four storeys, all dedicated to the work of Combine artists.'

'I bought a beautiful abstract piece for Jules's birthday last month,' Nathan says. 'It's transformed our kitchen. There's a duality to Combine art that doesn't exist in an ordinary painting. You're an artist, aren't you, Laurie-Amelia? We'll get you signed up for art therapy. It would be so exciting if your work sold.'

We glance behind us to check on Lara-Jay, but all we see is their back. We watch as Eliza gently leads them towards the apartment blocks.

Our Passing has been scheduled for next week. Nathan flushed with excitement when he delivered the news. 'You've now been out of your apartment for fourteen days,' he said, 'and you've coped incredibly well. My request was granted immediately. That's not a guarantee, Laurie-Amelia. More often than not, the initial Passing request is turned down.' He noticed our concerned expression. 'It's a milestone. You're emotionally ready to witness the burial. Aren't you excited?'

We're unsure how he's determined we're emotionally ready for this. It can't be based on our behaviour. Just yesterday, we hid under the bed and refused to come out. When Nathan crawled beneath to inject us, we screamed and kicked, our foot meeting his nose. He cried out. 'Laurie-Amelia,' he said, covering his bleeding nose with his hand. 'Calm down.' But we couldn't. 'He'll hurt us,' we shouted. 'He'll hurt us like he hurts her.'

Noah-Lucas stops by the apartment, a brief visit before their music therapy session. They mention picking up the trombone again, being surprised at how their skill hasn't faded. 'If anything,' they say, 'I might be even better now.' It's a shock to them; they had anticipated resistance. After all, Noah had been quite vocal about his feelings towards playing in big band.

Our therapy is art. No matter how tangled our thoughts or heavy our frustration, we find the motivation to get out of bed and make it to the art block in time for the class. Like Noah-Lucas's music, painting still comes naturally to us – all the better because we're both a part of it. When we paint, we connect in a way that's difficult to describe. There's no head-talk, no need to propose ideas, debate technique or worry about how the other is feeling. When we're painting, we think together, move together and create together. Only once the piece is complete do we step back and notice the differences: the brushstrokes that are a little looser, the palette slightly brighter, the forms less rigid than we're used to. It's a new rhythm, a new style now there are two minds at work during its creation.

Callie and Nathan are chatting on the sofa, discussing our Passing arrangements, pallbearers and gowns, that sort of thing. We sit on the footstool, watching Noah-Lucas. They're lying on their stomach on the lounge carpet, sorting through pieces of the jigsaw we started and abandoned. We realised, too late, that we should have looked for the edge pieces first and made the frame.

'Wasn't your Passing scary?' we ask. 'I hate the idea of being at my own funeral.'

'It's not a funeral,' Noah-Lucas says.

We frown, watching as they arrange the puzzle pieces by colour, carefully sorting through the pinks. It's what Nathan keeps telling us, but we don't buy it. *My body is being put underground. Mary is coming to say goodbye. How is that not a funeral?*

'It's not morbid like a funeral. It's not about a life ending, but a new one beginning. If anything, it's reaffirming. Who's your Witness?'

'Mary.'

A part of us was desperate for our Witness to be Albie, but we knew what the right decision was. We are permitted one Witness, and Mary is the correct choice. She deserves the closure, the chance to say goodbye to the body of her friend who was by her side for so many years.

Mary will be more level-headed at the Passing. She'll ensure everyone at home knows we're safe and well. Albie would struggle. He'd allow his views to influence his perspective. And he'd want an explanation. He'd want to know why we went through with this, what made us sure merging was the answer, and we wouldn't have anything to tell him.

We smile, imagining our reunion with Mary. It's something we like to think about whenever we're struggling to sleep. Every time, the imagining starts off so well. Mary's there, smiling, skipping towards us. She's so pleased, thrilled that we merged. But no matter how well the scene begins, it always ends the same way, with Mary dissolving in our arms.

Noah-Lucas is delighted by our smile, even after it fades. 'See,' they say. 'It *is* exciting. Even Lara-Jay enjoyed their Passing. You should have seen their face when they were reunited with Kath. It's the only time I've seen them happy.'

We watch as Noah-Lucas arranges the pink edge pieces in a neat row. *Do you think it was both of them who were happy? If I were unhappy, but you were excited, we'd still smile, wouldn't we? It's impossible to know which one of us is smiling.*

We worry about Lara-Jay a lot. We try not to, but we can't help it. Every time we see them, they seem so frail. Nathan gets frustrated by our concern. 'Lara-Jay is fine, Laurie-Amelia,' he always says. 'As I keep telling you, all Combines react to their Merge in a unique way. Please listen to me. Stop comparing their progress to yours and accept that Lara-Jay is doing just fine. It's disrespectful to their journey to keep judging them like this.'

We try not to judge, but it's difficult. It's been two weeks of walks and holistic sessions with Lara-Jay. Two weeks of us talking at them, rambling on in the hope of lifting their spirits. They're yet to acknowledge us beyond the occasional glance. Whenever we think we might be getting somewhere, that they might be about to speak, Eliza intervenes, interrupts, tells us Lara-Jay is getting tired, and insists they head back home.

Noah-Lucas begins sorting through the white puzzle pieces, lining up the straight edges just as they did with the pinks. They hold a piece up to the light, carefully checking it for patterns or markings.

'Do you worry about Lara-Jay?' we ask.

Noah-Lucas shakes their head. 'You know what Lara-Jay's like. Think of how much sulking Lara did, how angry she was at Jay, and how frustrated Jay was by her. Now imagine being trapped together, bickering twenty-four-seven. They've got to get used to each other. That's all. It must be really tough for them. Even I've had my fair share of internal disagreements.'

We raise our eyebrows. 'Really?'

'Oh yeah. Like the other day, I was remembering a really happy time to help myself fall asleep. That's what I like to do, remember happy moments and drift off peacefully. But that night, I kept arguing with myself about the memory, seeing conflicting versions of it, and insisting it wasn't happy at all. It made me so angry.'

'Why don't you share how you got through it?' Callie suggests. 'You've developed a brilliant coping mechanism. It might be helpful for Laurie-Amelia to hear about it.'

'I've started writing it down in my diary.' Noah-Lucas rotates a puzzle piece and slots it into place. 'I write the memory in the middle of the page. The memory that caused the conflict the other night was of my – of Lucas's– fifteenth birthday. So, that's what I wrote: *Lucas's birthday.* Then I split the page in two.

'On one side, I write the facts from the happy perspective. Things like, *I was happy. Noah was healthy. The family was together. Ellie was there. Mum and Dad were paying attention to me. The candles that refused to go out made everyone laugh.* That sort of thing. Then, on the other side, I write the conflicting memories. *I knew it was going to be the last of*

Lucas's birthdays that I'd be alive for. Lucas wasn't aware that I was sick again. I had a fight with Dad, who said I was being selfish for not telling Lucas the truth. I locked myself in the bathroom and cried.

'Then I highlight the compatible memories, the ones that can coexist without too much conflict. For example, I was both happy and knew I was sick. Mum was paying attention to me, and Dad was being an arsehole. Then I decide that's the version I'll think of in the future. The blended reality.'

'That's very impressive,' Nathan says. 'You should share that, Noah-Lucas, with as many Combines as you can. It's a valuable technique.'

Noah-Lucas doesn't seem to mind us observing them as they work on the puzzle. We'd join in, but we don't have much energy today. The tablets and the bombardment of triggering memories have left us feeling a little flat, glazed, as though we're an observer. As though we can't be seen.

'What song is that?' Noah-Lucas asks. They've completed a small section of the puzzle, a pink and white shape that we know, from the box, will form part of the sky. 'You've got a nice voice, Laurie-Amelia. I didn't know that about you.'

We pause, momentarily lost. *What are they talking about, Mum?*

The humming. I was humming. Weren't you?

We blink, bewildered. We hum again to check it really was us – that part of us that has been silent until now. We point at Nathan. *Tell him. Tell him I'm the one doing this.*

'The other part of me is humming,' we say.

Nathan's eyes widen as we begin again. We work together, playing with the volume as though testing out a new radio, turning the dial left and right. Nathan and Callie cheer and clap like we're a performer on a stage. We laugh loudly, both of us together, throwing our head back. Noah-Lucas smiles from the floor. 'Keep going, Laurie-Amelia,' they say. 'Hum with everything you've got.'

Nathan sits at the head of the dining room table, his usual place for our therapy sessions. Where we sit, he always says, is up to us. When he's upset with us we opt for the chair furthest from him, but today we feel like being close to him, absorbing every modicum of his pride. We sit on the chair next to his.

Nathan rests his fingers together. 'How are you feeling physically, Laurie-Amelia?'

We consider how we are. Our pace has increased, and we feel mostly steady on our feet. In the weeks since we've been out of the apartment, we've only wobbled a couple of times. It's strange – although we move with more confidence, inside we're no different, no more certain in what we're doing or how we got here.

'Good,' we say. 'Like I'm making progress.'

Nathan looks at the walking stick propped against the table.

'I'd like to keep using it,' we say quickly. 'I know I don't need to, but it makes me feel safe.' There's something about possessing a sturdy piece of wood, having our hand tightly wrapped round the handle. One swift whack with the stick, and we could cause enough damage to escape from danger. We don't voice this thought. 'There's no need for a weapon, Laurie-Amelia,' Nathan would say. 'You're not in any danger.'

'Let's talk about your goals for the week. With your Passing coming up, it can be easy to get distracted. I urge you not to, Laurie-Amelia. I advise you to set a clear goal and achieve it. Have you any in mind?'

I know what I want.
I want it, too.

We nod. We have our goal. There's no resistance, no bickering. We're aligned in our desire. 'I'd like to help Lara-Jay. I'd like to get them humming.'

Nathan smiles, and a warm feeling of validation washes over us. 'You achieved a wonderful milestone today,' he says. 'I hope you're feeling proud of yourself. It was quite the breakthrough. How did it feel to make a sound together?'

You take this one, Mum. You tell him how it felt.

We try, so intensely that it brings on an ache behind our ears, but no words come.

I can't. Humming is all I have for now.

'It felt good,' we say. 'It's the first time I've felt as though talking will be possible. I doubted what you were saying before. But now I believe you, Nathan. I know that I'll get there.'

'That's wonderful, Laurie-Amelia. Believing,' he says, 'is half the battle.'

We make the short walk to Lara-Jay's building early the next day. We pass the allotment, where Combines busy themselves harvesting fresh vegetables and turning over the soil for new plantings. *It's so peaceful here. I've never fancied rural living, but perhaps this is what we enjoy now. We certainly seem calmer out here than in London. What do you think?*

A Combine is bent over, pulling out weeds, whistling as they work. *Maybe. Gardening still doesn't appeal to me, though. I'm too impatient.*

A pair of Combines pass us on bicycles, their Support Workers following behind, coasting down the hill. One of them lifts his feet off the pedals, grinning as he speeds up.

Oh, let's ask if we can cycle, Amelia. I haven't cycled in years. You know how your father felt about bikes. I never liked to get on one. It felt like a betrayal somehow. It doesn't feel that way anymore. Is that your influence, do you think?

We refrain from asking Nathan if we can cycle. We'll progress to the bikes when we're ready, but for now it's important we walk. Walking allows us to get our bearings. It gives us time to notice the smaller details: the emblems carved into the trunks of the trees, the birdhouses and feeders, perched high on the branches, and the security cameras, carefully camouflaged within the dense foliage.

'Why are there so many cameras?' we ask when we reach Lara-Jay's apartment block and spot a little red light hidden in the planter.

'They're there to keep you safe, Laurie-Amelia. Don't let the cameras worry you.'

But they do worry us. They feel intrusive, invading our privacy with their unblinking stare. The more we look for them, the more we find. There are cameras disguised as outdoor lights, discreetly positioned in the ceilings of buildings, concealed within signage. They seem to multiply, popping up in places we're certain they weren't before. We try to keep track, but it's so hard to remember.

We notice a red light in the planter, glowing among the foliage. *We already saw this one, Mum. Just now. Don't you remember?* Our legs begin to tingle, but we force the feeling away. It's natural to forget sometimes. Think of the positives. Find comfort in the cameras. It's a good thing we're being so closely observed.

Lara-Jay doesn't smile when they see us. We hug them, and they remain stiff. They're so rigid and cold, as though they're made of stone. Perhaps they are. It would explain why they walk so slowly, why it takes such effort to lift their feet.

We tuck our free arm into theirs and attempt to guide them forward, but they're resistant. 'How are you, Lara-Jay?' we ask. 'Have you had a good morning?'

They say nothing. It doesn't bother us; we knew they wouldn't. Nathan and Eliza fall into step behind us, trusting us to walk with Lara-Jay. We've got good at supporting them.

'I'm Passing next week,' we tell them quietly. 'I'm a bit nervous about it. Noah-Lucas said that Kath was your Witness. It must have been nice to see her again.'

We watch for any flicker of emotion, but they keep their gaze fixed ahead, revealing nothing. We take our usual route, walking slowly down the path towards the pond. We know we shouldn't, and a part of us doesn't want to, but another part of us yearns for it, desperate for a glimpse. *I can't bear the emotional toll that follows when he fades, Amelia. I wish you wouldn't give in to your desire so easily.*

We can turn back, Mum. Just say the word.

But the word never comes, so we continue walking.

Our longing to see Albie is growing by the day. We think of him almost constantly. For now, the hallucinations are all we have, and the pond seems to summon them. The high of seeing Albie, the euphoria of watching him feed the ducks, is worth the downturn when he disappears. Often we cry when it happens, and Nathan sighs as he wipes our tears. 'You can come back and feed the ducks tomorrow, Laurie-Amelia. You needn't cry.'

The path slopes gently downwards. Lara-Jay slows, as they always do. We hold on to them tightly. 'I've got you,' we say. 'There's no rush.'

We wait until the path levels out again, and we're nearing the pond, before trying again to get them to speak. 'Mary's going to be my Witness,' we say. 'I think she'll be a blubbering mess. I would be if I were Witnessing her burial. Nathan keeps saying it's a good thing, that I should be excited about it. But I'm not. I can't stand the thought of my body being trapped underground without its soul, watching as it's covered with soil, and seeing Mary grieve. There's a reason we don't host funerals while people are still alive to witness them. They're too painful, too raw. It's a reminder of everything we're losing, everything we're leaving behind.'

We keep talking, relentless Noah-Lucas-type chatter, until their arm relaxes in ours. When we finally reach the pond, we look around for Albie, but he's nowhere to be seen. We wait, but he doesn't appear. The disappointment is overwhelming. Our eyes sting. We grasp Lara-Jay for support. *Breathe, Amelia. It's because we have other things on our mind. If you want to see Albie badly enough, he'll turn up. You know he will. But there's something we want more. Let's do what we came for.*

A duck dips its head beneath the surface of the pond, searching for food. Tiny bubbles rise as it forages underwater.

'Do you remember that I struggle with talking, too, Lara-Jay? The Transfer part of me can't speak. It's frustrating and upsetting. I can't imagine how difficult it is for you being entirely mute. But you'll get there. I know you will.'

The duck's head resurfaces briefly before disappearing again. Ripples spread from the spot where the duck hunts, distorting the reflection of the trees on the water's surface. They twist and warp, unsteady and ephemeral.

We stand in silence for a while. Lara-Jay seems transfixed by the water, staring glassy-eyed at the reflections as they swell and shimmer. 'I started humming yesterday,' we tell them. 'The Transfer part of me, I mean. It finally happened. I finally made a noise. Would you like to hear?'

We hum quietly to a song Mitchell used to love. The words we haven't retained, but the rhythm remains. It rolls smoothly, like the ripples on the pond. *I think it was something about sailors. Something about being at sea.* Lara-Jay keeps their eyes on the water. We're certain they have no interest in our breakthrough, but when we stop they tap our arm, urging us to continue. We laugh, and our eyes sting again — not with disappointment this time, but relief. Lara-Jay *does* understand. They *do* hear us.

'Why don't you try, Lara-Jay? See if you can make any sound at all.'

Their eyes shift, becoming fixed on the path.

We've lost them. We were so close. What made them disappear? They heard, even enjoyed, our humming. Now, they're choosing to block us out.

A hot surge of anger flares through us. 'Lara-Jay, I know you can hear me. It's rude to ignore people.' Our voice rises, sharp and cutting. 'You're being rude. Look at me.'

To our surprise, they do.

They move their head slowly, and their vacant gaze eventually lands on us.

We look into their eyes, properly, for the first time since

their Merge. And finally, we see them. All of them. The panic in their stare.

Lara. Trapped. Silenced.

She stares with such intensity, such desperation, that we hear her unspoken words. We know what she wants. We know who she's searching for. She always found such comfort in us.

In me.

In Laurie.

And now she needs to see us, to know she's okay, that she can do this, that she can exist happily inside her father. *But I can't tell her. I have no voice. How can she believe I'm here when I can't tell her myself?*

We take Lara-Jay's hand. Ours feels so small in theirs, so unable to provide the comfort we need it to. *Go on, Mum. Do it.*

We close our eyes and hum gently, a low note that vibrates in our throat. We think of Lara, of how much she relied on us to get her through. We see her, in the rare moments she felt joy, her shy smile. She needs us. She needs me.

Our humming gains momentum, and then morphs into something more.

Something real.

Our voice escapes effortlessly, as though it has a will of its own.

'I'm here,' we whisper. 'It's me. It's Lor.'

Then Lara-Jay is crying, and their tears become contagious. Neither of us makes a sound or breaks the gaze. We're silent in our shared grief. We mourn together. Our bodies. Our autonomy. Our selves.

Lara-Jay grips our hands, their nails digging into our palms. Their tears fall faster.

'Tell me,' we whisper. 'Please, Lara-Jay, let me help you.'

'Lor?'

We stare, taken aback by the sound of their voice, the apparent ease with which they've spoken. 'Yes,' we say. 'It's Lor. It's me.'

They touch our face, wiping away our tears. They attempt a smile, but it's met with a shaky exhale. 'You're really in there?'

'Yes.'

They close their eyes, their chin quivering.

'What is it?' we say again, together, united. 'What's wrong?'

'She's not here,' they whisper. 'Lara's not here.'

The gown we've been provided with is silk. It reminds us of the bridesmaid dress we wore to Mary's wedding. We worried it was too revealing with its almost invisible straps, but Mary assured us it was perfect. 'I designed it specially,' she said. 'It was made just for you.'

Her wedding was held in a small, weathered church on the coast of Cornwall. Besides family, Mitchell and I were the only guests – two witnesses to the intimate ceremony. Afterwards, we gathered on the beach for the wedding breakfast, our toes sinking into the sand as we ate. As evening fell, we wrapped ourselves in thick blankets, watching the setting sun, sharing in Mary and Stuart's happiness as the horizon sank into the sea.

We wonder if Mary will have the same thoughts when she sees us. If the sight of us in this gown will take her back.

Eliza styles our hair, singing softly as she brushes. We watch her in the mirror as she secures the bun with an elegant green hairpin. Two tendrils of hair have been left to frame our face in delicate curls. 'What do you think?' Eliza holds a small mirror behind us to show us the finished look. Our hair is twisted tightly into a neat ring. Below the bun is our tattoo. We run our finger over the mandala, following the gentle curve of the loose 's' that splits the design, feeling the subtle rise of ink beneath our skin. We'd forgotten it was there.

All those months we spent discussing what tattoo to get to mark my sixtieth. We couldn't agree on anything. Perhaps we were destined to wait for this one. Now we have a tattoo that truly belongs to the both of us. I like it, don't you? It's prettier than I remembered, more delicate.

'I love it,' we say. 'Thank you, Eliza.' Even if we didn't approve of her styling, we'd never admit it. We can't argue against the traditional hairstyle for the Passing, not after Eliza spent so long ensuring the bun was exactly right, symmetrical and of even thickness. She puts the little mirror on the bed and squeezes our shoulders, her eyes meeting ours.

She'll be the one officiating today, leading the burial. A privilege, she keeps saying. An honour to be involved in the next stage of our journey.

'Is Lara-Jay coming to my Passing?' we ask. 'Did you tell them how much I want to see them?'

Eliza begins collecting up the hairpins and combs, putting them in a little purple pouch. 'I did tell them how much their presence would mean to you, but I can't promise anything. They haven't been out since that walk to the pond.' She picks up a can of hairspray and begins shaking it. 'Close your eyes, Laurie-Amelia. And cover your mouth.'

We think back to the last time we saw Lara-Jay. When they dropped to their knees and cried, their cheek pressed against the gravel, the stones imprinted on their skin. 'I can't hear her,' they sobbed, tears wetting the stones. 'Why can't I hear her?'

We crouched beside them, resting a hand on their cheek. Their face was hot despite the cold air. 'What do you mean you can't hear her?'

Then Nathan and Eliza were pulling Lara-Jay to their feet, hoisting them up with their hands under their armpits. Lara-Jay rose like a mannequin being repositioned in a shop window. No struggle, no resistance. They closed their eyes, relinquishing all control. Eliza took charge, lifting their arm and draping it over her shoulders. 'What do you mean you can't hear her?' we asked again. 'Aren't you having any head-talk?'

Lara-Jay kept their eyes closed but shook their head.

'None? Nothing at all?'

'Enough, Laurie-Amelia,' Nathan warned, his hand still under Lara-Jay's arm. 'You can see they're distressed. Drop it.'

'But—'

'Enough!'

We jumped. Nathan never raised his voice. Not even when we failed the tests.

Eliza stroked Lara-Jay's hand as she walked them slowly back to their apartment. She spoke soothingly the whole time, assuring Lara-Jay that everything was all right, that the head-talk would return, that this was nothing to worry about. 'You spoke,' she kept saying. 'You found your voice, Lara-Jay. Let's focus on that remarkable achievement.'

As we walked home, we considered how strange it was that our voice had arrived along with Lara-Jay's, how our first words formed just moments before theirs. We thought of their panicked eyes searching ours, of Lara trapped inside, desperately looking for someone who could see her.

Since then, we've spent countless hours dissecting the reasons behind Lara's silence, arguing over which theory seems most plausible: Is it the unresolved conflict between them? Or because Lara refused to fully engage in the sessions designed to bring them closer? Or is it something more sinister? Is Lara deliberately tormenting Jay, refusing to speak? Hiding within him, sulking, intent on driving him mad?

Anxiety swells as we make our way to the church, growing like the dark clouds overhead. Nathan holds a large umbrella, the rain pattering on its canopy. We remain close to him, our gown bunched in our hands to keep it from spoiling on the wet gravel path. We tread carefully, not wanting to slip. We've no walking stick; Nathan insisted we left it behind.

Combines and Support Workers offer smiles and congratulations as we pass. Some bow their heads. 'From what was,' they say, 'we emerge anew.'

We nod our thanks, our voice faltering, our mouth dry. Nathan speaks for us, delivering the expected response. 'Our past we honour, our future we embrace. In the Merge, we protect our place.'

The hymns have begun. Their tones, carried by the wind, wrap themselves around us, threatening to suffocate. We concentrate on our breathing, taking large gulps of air. A fish stranded on land.

Combines spill out of the church, a sea of green suits and gowns. Anyone with hair long enough to be tied up sports the same bun. So many have turned up to watch us Pass. We knew they would. It was the same for Noah-Lucas and Lara-Jay. Everyone wants to witness the burial of the experimental Combines, to say they were there for this moment in history.

The rain grows heavier. Umbrellas are raised, popping up like fireworks.

We manage a smile as we pass through the gaggle of Combines loitering outside the church. Each one bows their head respectfully.

The church, though built for The Village, has the appearance of a building centuries old, its rough weathered stone mottled with moss and lichen. Nathan folds the umbrella, shaking it vigorously to remove the wet. We tighten our grip on his arm. 'You're a pioneer, Laurie-Amelia,' he says quietly. 'You're going to change the world.'

We walk slowly down the aisle. Merged faces, half man, half woman, are carved on the end of each pew.

I've never liked churches. Not since I was forced to attend one every Sunday as a little girl.

At the altar, a sculpture of steel and stone depicts two figures locked in an eternal embrace. Behind them is a large stained-glass window. In the centre stands Our Combine, head raised, hands splayed wide. Encircling it are smaller panels displaying the mandala. There's a pulpit and lit white candles, but no cross. How strange it seems to celebrate the

Passing in a church, when the Christians were so vocal in their outrage. Their warnings were clear: life is a gift from God, not to be tampered with by mortal hands.

The memory floods in.

The chaos of the streets. The furious faces of the activists, their fists raised in defiance. We're among them, shouting, fury in our hearts. The weight of the placard, held high above us. The fear – the terror – that we'd be ignored.

The church comes back into focus. We're halfway down the aisle, nearing the altar.

The statue. The candles.

It wasn't just Christians who condemned the Merge. All faiths stood united – Muslims, Jews, Hindus, Buddhists, Sikhs. The solidarity transcended religious differences. Religious leaders stood side by side, denouncing the Merge as a violation of divine order and human dignity. We knew, we were certain, that merging was wrong. And now, here we are, a Combine, about to Pass.

A chill sweeps over us. *Do you remember the protests? We were so sure, so certain—*

A clammy hand grips our arm.

We recognise the sapphire ring. The mole under the middle knuckle. We stop. But before we can react, Nathan lifts Mary's hand from our arm and pulls us away. 'Don't be distracted,' he says. 'Remember to curtsey when you're in front of the statue.'

We glance back. So many unfamiliar faces. Mary stands among them, a solitary figure dressed in white amidst the purple and green. We reach the statue, curtsey deeply, holding tightly to Nathan for support.

We turn. Noah-Lucas smiles at us from the front pew.

Then we see them. Lara-Jay.

They came.

They're standing, allowing us to slide in between them and Noah-Lucas. We touch their hand. 'Thank you,' we whisper. 'I'm so pleased you're here.'

They nod, eyes downcast.

We sit, and Noah-Lucas squeezes our knee, smiling encouragingly. We look back at Mary. We hadn't considered before now what a big ask this was. She'll have undergone interviews and background checks to be granted access to The Village, and now she has to sit silently among strangers and watch her best friend's burial.

'Look forward,' Noah-Lucas whispers. 'Don't torture yourself. Watching won't make it arrive any faster.' We realise they mean the coffin. The body. My body. We don't want to watch.

Mary wipes her eyes. We turn away. We know how she feels. We've been where she is, crying in a cold church.

Our mind drifts back to all those Sundays forced to sit on the hard pew. Forced to stand for the hymns and listen as he prayed. *In my experience, the people who spend their time preaching about loving and being kind to others are often the cruellest individuals. The good people, the people who would never think to do otherwise, don't feel kindness is something that needs to be taught. It's the people who preach about being a good person, Amelia. They're the worst ones out there.*

We shift position, trying to prevent the memory that threatens to rise. *We never once sat at the front. He preferred us to be at the back where we couldn't be seen. He could get away with anything. Hidden, even under the eye of God. I always felt so squashed, as little as I was.*

Then we're back there, sitting in a large, echoing church, squeezed in beside him. His leg is against ours, and he stinks of stale smoke. We want to move away, to escape the smell, but we don't dare. We stroke the kneeler hanging in front of our knees, tracing the pattern of red crosses, trying to distract ourselves from the feeling of his hand on our leg.

There's a harp playing now, and everyone's standing. We're the only one still sitting, gripping the edge of the pew, our face hot. There's a tap on our shoulder. Lara-Jay. We blink up at them, and they put their thumb up, a question in their eyes: *All okay?*

We nod, get to our feet and force a smile. 'Yes,' we say quietly. 'Thank you. How are you?' We mirror their gesture, putting our thumb up. A new theory comes to us: What if Jay is silencing Lara? What if what Lara's saying, deep inside, is simply too painful for him to process, so he's blocking her out, refusing to let her voice break through?

Eliza appears, her deep-purple robe brushing the floor.

We catch our breath, then find we can't breathe at all. We're emptied of air, leaving our lungs hollow, as though we've been struck square in the chest. The coffin is here, being carried by pallbearers we don't recognise. Their faces are solemn, their gowns purple. Support Workers. They've the expression of people carrying the weight of a corpse: dead.

We force ourselves to breathe, gasping for air, inhaling as much as our lungs can hold. Someone clings to our hand, gripping tightly.

The coffin makes its slow journey towards the altar.

We're in there.

Dead. Decomposing to dust and bones.

A cry escapes us. We cover our mouth.

Another memory. The first time we met. Skin on skin. One of us terrified of the bright new world, the other trembling with love.

That love poured into our lives like a flood, unstoppable and overwhelming.

Now, that love is gone.

There will be no more hugs. No more leaning into Mum's

embrace, feeling as though we could remain there, safely wrapped in her arms, forever. No more seeing her eyes light up when she laughs, the genuine joy spreading effortlessly to everyone around her. We'll never again sit across from her, sipping tea and sharing stories, her gaze always so gentle and curious.

The surge of grief takes us out like a punch. We fall backwards onto the pew.

Lara-Jay leans close. 'I found it helped to close my eyes,' they whisper. Again, it seems so effortless, so natural for them to be speaking. 'There's no rule that says you have to watch.'

The coffin reaches the front of the church. We watch through half-closed eyes. There's a powerful need in us to witness this moment, to see it in order to believe it. It's like watching ourselves be put down, seeing the injection, the needle, a fine strand of hair, sliding in, and watching life quickly ebb away, like something physical leaving the room.

Someone cries loudly behind us, another barely containing their grief. Mary. We don't turn. Our eyes remain on the coffin.

Mum. Me. Us.

Drenched in darkness. A body in a casket. Blood siphoned away. Our face made up, unreal as a mask. Grotesque.

We know, somewhere deep down, too far to reach, that this isn't what it appears. It's not like Dad. Not like Mitchell. This isn't death, just the disposal of a body, not of a person. But the grief, it turns out, remains the same.

Once the service is complete, we move outside. The weather has worsened. The umbrella proves useless. It blows inside out, its spokes buckling. The wind drives the rain into our face. 'Just here, Laurie-Amelia.' Nathan's chin is tucked to his chest, his eyes squinting against the rain.

We stop beside a deep hole.

Bile rises in our throat. We swallow hard, trying to regain control. *It's only a body we're burying. A vessel, nothing more.* To the left of the hole is a large mound of soil. Too much soil. Enough for three graves at least. We imagine it piling on top of the coffin, the earth closing in around it, the dirt pressing in from all sides, squeezing out any remaining breath.

We take a step back, concentrate on the feeling of our gown, soaked through despite the jacket we've been provided with. The silk clings uncomfortably to our skin, and we will the weight of it to ground us like an anchor. It doesn't work. Our breathing has become laboured, our lungs failing to function.

We take another step back. There are hundreds of gravestones surrounding us, each one perfectly kept. Beyond the graves is untouched land, ready to accommodate more Transfer bodies, the Host bodies left to grieve.

We stumble, lightheaded. Then Mary is there, standing between us and our grave. Her wet hair clings to her face. 'Breathe,' she says. 'Breathe with me like we used to.'

Her hands take ours.

We'd sit with Mary after Mitchell died, both of us together. She'd hold each of our hands. We'd breathe. We'd recover. Not die, like he had. Not die, like we thought we were about to. We do the same now, using her breaths as our guide. 'Good,' she says. 'That's better.' She takes another breath, long and deep. The wind pushes between us, trying to separate us. But Mary won't let go.

'I need proof, Lor,' she says. 'I need to know you're really in there. Now's the time. Now's the time to prove to me it's you.' She moves closer, until her face is just inches from ours. 'Tell me what was written on that piece of paper.'

We close our eyes and hum gently. We think of the slip of paper, the words scribbled onto it. The code that was so important. The one that proved...

When we open our eyes, Mary is there, searching our face. 'Lor?'

We nod. 'I'm here,' we whisper. 'I'm here, you silly sod.'

Mary holds us so tightly that it's impossible to move. 'Thank god,' she whispers. 'Thank god, thank god, thank god.'

By the time Eliza begins addressing us, the rain has stopped. Only the wind remains. It carries her voice across the graveyard and leaves us shaking, our teeth clicking together as she raises her hands to the sky. 'Today we gather here to celebrate the progression of Laurie Evelyn Anderson, our beloved Transfer, who has sacrificed her body to ensure the existence of many tomorrows.' The pallbearers emerge from the church, bringing with them our coffin. 'As we prepare to lower the coffin into the earth, we must remember that this is a joyous occasion. This is sacrifice in its purest, most transcendental form. Laurie's body is being returned to the earth, and her legacy will live on for all eternity. Her previous, precious vessel will remain sacred, protected in the heart of The Village forever more.'

Eliza steps back and the pallbearers approach the grave.

We watch as they lower the casket into the earth, using thick green ribbon to support the weight. Once it has safely reached the bottom, the bearers extract the ribbons and begin to twirl them, creating a series of elaborate shapes. 'Mary, Laurie-Amelia's chosen Witness, will now come forward and bid farewell to the beloved body of Laurie Evelyn Anderson.'

The dance continues, the green ribbons pirouetting around us as Mary approaches to say goodbye. She takes our hand, tears flowing freely. 'You *knew*, Lor. And you, Amelia. You both knew this would work. I'm sorry for doubting you, for trying to talk you out of it. I'm so happy you've done this, that your memories will be preserved, that *you* will be preserved.' She hugs us and we hold her gently, both of us shivering in the cold. 'Well done. Well done for being so brave.'

'I love you, Mary.'

She doesn't dissolve as in our dreams but kisses us on the cheek before moving to the mound of dirt. She takes a handful of sticky soil and tosses it onto the coffin, lowers her head. 'Thank you for your sacrifice.'

Support Workers and Combines, some we've met, many we haven't, come forward to thank us and cover the coffin with soil. When Noah-Lucas approaches, it's we who reach for them, it's we who long to share in their acceptance. 'You've done it,' they say, their cheeks reddened by the cold. 'You've actually done it, Laurie-Amelia. You should be so proud.' They bring us in for a hug, placing their hand gently on the back of our neck, cupping our mandala. A feeling of calm washes over us.

I think we can do this. If we really try, we can make a good life as a Combine, do as Mary said, preserve our precious memories and continue to thrive. We can get back to our life.

We break apart and Noah-Lucas lowers their head. There's no need for them to thank us for our sacrifice, but they do. We watch as they move to the mound of soil and take a handful. *Such lovely boys.* We think of Noah, how he'd never have coped in this cold weather. He wouldn't have had the strength.

We're smiling properly for the first time, and they're smiling too.

But as they approach the coffin, preparing to sprinkle the dirt, there's a cry.

Noah-Lucas's smile falters, the dirt still clutched in their hands. Their eyes widen as they look around, unsure where the cry came from.

Another cry. We turn to see a Combine in the crowd pointing at the church, their arm stiff with urgency. Confusion ripples through the group. More hands are pointing in the same direction, and the murmurs grow louder. Gasps. Frantic whispers. A Support Worker suddenly breaks into a run, sprinting towards the church, shouting at the top of his lungs. It's Nathan.

We squint, struggling to see what everyone is staring at.

A figure is perched on the bell tower, one hand gripping the wall, their legs dangling over the edge.

We move closer.

The figure lets go of the wall, their arms spreading wide like wings.

'No!' someone shouts. 'Hold on! Help is on the way!'

The crowd erupts into a frenzy of shouts and desperate pleas. The figure is wearing green – a Combine – but we can't quite—

'Oh my god.' Noah-Lucas's voice trembles, then rises, panicked. 'Oh my god!' The earth slips from their hands as they sprint past us, arms flailing. 'Lara-Jay!' they scream. 'Lara-Jay, it's me! It's me, Noah-Lucas. Lara—'

But it's too late. Lara-Jay jumps.

A single, haunting scream splits the air as they fall.

Whenever we close our eyes, we see Lara-Jay plummet. For a moment, the wind seems to hold and support them, then their arms flail and their hands claw at nothing. There's the scream. Then the soft, almost liquid impact of their body breaking into pieces on the gravel. We feel the tiny razor-edged stones embedding themselves into our exposed skin.

It's us diving into oblivion.

We're wrapped in a towel, shivering on the edge of the bed. Nathan's trying to cajole us into getting dressed. We took a long cold shower to focus our attention away from the image of Lara-Jay's buckled, disassembled body. It didn't work.

Nathan perches beside us. We watch in the mirror as he speaks, aware of the cadence of his voice, but not his words.

Lara-Jay's body flashes before us. Human origami.

We must scream, because Nathan is hushing us, gently shaking us, his eyes bloodshot. 'It is not your fault,' he says desperately. 'Please don't cry. There was nothing you could have done. You wouldn't blame Noah-Lucas, would you? Or Benjamin-Annie. It would be nonsensical. It's just as unfair to blame yourself.'

'Benjamin-Annie?' we manage to say.

It's so rare that they're mentioned. Nathan doesn't ever speak about them unless we press him directly, and even then we're met with a reprimand. 'You know the rules, Laurie-Amelia,' he always reminds us. 'Benjamin-Annie is entitled to their privacy. Their progress isn't mine to share.'

'They're okay, Laurie-Amelia. Angela's looking after them.'

'I want to see them.'

'I know you do, but I'm afraid you can't. No one is allowed out of their apartments. The Village is in lockdown. You know this.'

'We're a support group, Nathan. You brought us together, made us a family, told us to lean on each other. And now, when it matters most, you force us apart. It makes no sense.'

'To you,' he says, 'maybe not. But we're the experts, Laurie-Amelia. We know what's best for Combines. And moving from your residence before you've had time to properly mourn and process Lara-Jay's death most certainly is *not* what's best.'

'Lara was always so miserable,' we say. 'She never hid how much she hated her dad. And Jay made no secret of how difficult he found her. Why did you let them merge?'

Nathan sighs, rubbing a hand over his face. 'Their compatibility scores were incredibly high. There was no indication their Merge would be any more challenging than anyone else's.'

We frown. It was obvious – to us, to everyone – that they would struggle the most. Even Nathan said how much further they had to go, how much unresolved conflict they were carrying with them.

Nathan smiles, a painful, unnatural expression. 'I have some good news for you.' His smile widens further, a wound being forced open. 'Mary was so delighted by your successful Merge and how well you seemed at your Passing that she decided to merge herself. She asked us to find her a match, and we did. A perfect match. Her name is Maisie, and she's twenty-three. Mary was delighted by the age, thinking Amelia would have loved her. She said the two of you would be brilliant Combine friends, that you could relive your twenties together. You inspired her, Laurie-Amelia. Even in the wake of such a tragedy, your inspiration reached her. I think that speaks volumes about how well you're doing. She's starting her Preparation Period as early as next month. Isn't it wonderful?'

Mary's merging? We'll both be in our twenties again... Girls together? Am I understanding this correctly, Amelia?

It's too much to digest. The bedroom melts, and suddenly Nathan is replaced by two officers, one male and one female, standing on our doorstep. We're fourteen, wearing our Tweetie pyjamas and staring at them blankly. We don't say anything, don't respond when the male officer asks if Mrs Anderson is home. We just stand there, silent and motionless.

'Who is it, Amelia?' Mum calls. 'Tell whoever it is I'll be with them in a second.'

'My mum's coming,' we say.

Then we're not Amelia, but Laurie. We're on the phone, telling Mary there's someone at the door and apologising for not answering her questions. Amelia looks so tiny standing beside the two officers, who've stepped into, and blocked, the hallway. We see the seriousness of their expressions. 'What's wrong?' we ask, the phone clutched tightly in our hand.

'Mrs Anderson?' The female officer looks mildly shocked. We're accustomed to such a reaction; we don't look old enough to be married to Mitchell, much more likely to be his daughter.

'Why don't you go to your room, sweetheart,' the male officer's saying, gently pushing Amelia towards the stairs. 'So we can have a word with your mother in private.'

We drape our arm protectively round Amelia's shoulders.

'What's wrong? What's happened?'

'I'm afraid there's been an accident, Mrs Anderson. Your husband, Mitchell Anderson, has been involved in a terrible accident.'

We're fourteen again, watching Mum collapse, hitting her head on the wall before she reaches the floor. We don't help or comfort her. We leave that to the officers, just as we left Lara-Jay to Eliza and Nathan the day they opened up to us.

The gravel dug into their flesh that day too, and we allowed it to happen. We didn't scoop them up, didn't brush the stones from their cheek, didn't hold them close and tell them it was going to be okay.

A voice breaks through. 'Laurie-Amelia, what can you smell? Take a nice deep breath and tell me what you can smell.' There are hands on our shoulders, leading us gently back into the room. 'Come on, Laurie-Amelia. Tell me. What can you smell?'

We inhale. There's a subtle fragrance, crisp and fresh. 'Washed bedlinen,' we say. 'And – eucalyptus.'

'Good. That's very good, Laurie-Amelia. What about textures? Really concentrate. What can you feel?'

We run our palms over the soft surface. 'A duvet.'

'Very good. You're in your bedroom, in your apartment. Are things coming back into focus? There's nothing here to be afraid of. You're perfectly safe.' There's a man, Nathan, sitting beside us. On his lap is a red bag, which we know contains the injection needed to sedate us. The bag is zipped shut and our arm doesn't ache. We must have recovered on our own.

'He's dead?' we whisper.

'*They*, yes,' Nathan says. 'Lara-Jay is dead.'

Lara-Jay.

The tears come again.

We're eighteen, sitting on the floor in the lime-green bathroom, our back against the cold radiator. Our mother is in the bathtub, one arm hanging limply over the edge, her slit wrist just inches from the bloodstained tiles. The steam's not enough to soften the image. The blood glows, unnaturally red.

Is that how she died, Mum? Did she hurt herself? Like Lara-Jay?

We feel the needle this time. And we give in to its sweet relief.

The Village has been opened to reporters. We stand at the living room window, observing their procession along the gravel paths. They wear fluorescent tabards, the type worn by road cyclists and equestrians. In place of BUILD CYCLE LANES or PLEASE PASS WIDE AND SLOW is the word PRESS. There's no sign of a camera; they must be stashed in the heavy military-looking bags they're carrying, this slow, silent army moving beneath us.

Remember how much Dad hated cyclists? It takes a while for the memory to crystallise. That's how it's been since Nathan altered our medication again. Memories assemble themselves slowly until the pictures are finally complete. We smile, remembering Mitchell's aversion to middle-aged men in Lycra. It was the only trivial thing that truly riled him. 'Fucking idiots,' he'd say as we crawled along behind the bikes jostling for position. 'Cycling in the middle of the fucking road as though they fucking own it.' We'd smile at each other, biting the inside of our cheeks to prevent laughter. His voice was too soft for his insults. We always waited until the journey was over, until we were safely out of the car and he was out of earshot. Then we'd giggle about his profanity. *He always seemed so gentle until he got behind the wheel of a car, didn't he?*

The journalists are being escorted through the complex by men and women wearing black. Regular people. Important people. They must be; why else would they be trusted with such a role? 'Who are these people?' we ask, watching as a pair of women enter an apartment block.

'Village Representatives,' Nathan says. His watch beeps, and so does ours. 'How are the visions today?'

We nod. 'Better.'

The image of Lara-Jay falling from the bell tower hasn't haunted us since Nathan switched our medication. We're experiencing hardly any hallucinations at all. It's saving us, but Nathan is concerned. 'I'm worried about the impact the medication's adjustment is having on you,' he said earlier, when we opened the door to him and didn't immediately register who we were looking at. We stepped back in alarm. 'I know you don't cope well with the hallucinations, Laurie-Amelia, but it's crucial that we find a balance between managing your symptoms and ensuring that you're not too detached from reality.'

We shook our head, panic fluttering through us. Since Lara-Jay's death, the new medication is the only thing holding us together. We need to stay numbed, dulled, in order to cope. 'Please keep me on it a little while longer. I'll do better, Nathan. I'll be more present. I promise I will.'

'Good,' Nathan says now. 'We'll keep going with these meds for today. It's not such a bad idea to be a little hazy with all the chaos that will be going on out there.' He leaves the room to fetch our pills. We watch as a 'Village Representative' escorts a group of reporters towards the library. One of the journalists is tall and slim, with blond curls. Our heart lurches, and we bang on the glass. We go to shout, to call out to him. Then we catch a glimpse of the man's profile. It's not Albie. It never is.

Desperation tightens in our chest; we need to hear Albie's voice, to draw strength from his steadiness. His resolve. He'd know what to do. He'd have a plan for coping without Lara-Jay, a way to ensure their death was not in vain.

Our banging has got the attention of another journalist. She looks up, smiles and waves. We stare down at her. We're supposed to wave back, to be welcoming, to show her how delightful life is here in The Village. The announcement that woke us this morning instructed us to *approach the day with enthusiasm and openness.* We stared at the faint spiral pattern on the ceiling through narrowed eyes.

The morning announcements used to be a source of comfort, a gentle nudge to start the day with a positive outlook. We'd listen to the affirmations, and they'd infuse us with strength and reassurance. Now, they feel hollow. Recycled platitudes designed to distract us from the cracks in the system, to prevent us from seeing the truth: that Lara and Jay were told, repeatedly, that everything was fine. The Support Workers encouraged – no, *forced* – an addict to merge, and then blamed their addiction when it all went wrong. That's what we've been told: Lara-Jay killed themselves because of their inability to be reliable and honest.

'I'm afraid we've discovered that Lara was dishonest during her compatibility tests,' Nathan told us a few days ago. 'I know this is difficult to hear, especially considering how close you were. It's painful to learn that you've been deceived. But it appears that Lara and Jay's scoring was inaccurate due to her – falsehoods.' He shook his head. 'No one could have known. Addicts are notoriously untrustworthy, and unfortunately she has proven herself to be no exception.'

A smiling 'Village Representative', a suited man with red hair, is looking up at us now, his hand shielding his eyes from the sun. Of course the sun's shining today.

Nathan escorts us to Eliza's interview, where our presence is required to show the world's press that the experiment remains on track. The majority of the residents stay inside. We look up and see them watching from their apartment windows, a frieze of pale faces. Three storeys up, a Combine with a female appearance has their palms splayed against the pane.

We pass a cluster of Combines whispering excitedly. The lucky few trusted to be outside. Those with long hair have it tied in buns, their tattoos proudly displayed for the cameras. Their Support Workers loiter nearby, smiling as we pass.

'You do remember how to conduct yourself with people from the outside?' Nathan asks as we cross the courtyard, where the reporters are gathered, their cameras now slung round their necks. We look at him, our eyebrows raised. He nods. 'Sorry. Of course you do.'

Since the press day was announced last week, we've had this etiquette drilled into us. Each morning, we wake to reminders of how crucial it is to leave a lasting impression. Variations of the same message: *As we prepare for the arrival of the world's press, remember to embody the values of resilience and positivity that define every resident here in The Village. Your actions in the coming days will profoundly shape the perception of Combines everywhere. May you inspire non-Combines around the world to merge and protect humanity from itself. Failure to do so will reflect poorly on all of us and result in necessary adjustments to your current freedoms.*

The threat is veiled but clear: if we fall short, if we present anything less than perfection, we'll lose our privileges. We'll be confined to our apartments again, forced to spend endless days alone.

'It's bullshit,' we said to Nathan. 'This isn't how you rehabilitate people. You don't threaten to take their freedom if they express their feelings. People are mourning. They're scared. They want answers. That's not a crime.'

'Careful, Laurie-Amelia.' He glanced at the door of our apartment, closed and locked, the chain securely fastened. 'If you're heard speaking like that, you'll be spending time inside.'

The imposition of draconian rules, fed to us through the announcements, has made The Village feel emptier with each passing day. Fewer Combines are outside, while more and more faces press against the windows, watching from behind the glass.

It feels most unsettling after sunset when the curtains are drawn, casting shadows that shift and flicker. Occasionally, a Combine peers out, observing us as we pass by. Each time, we check to see if it's Benjamin-Annie. It never is.

Nathan's been growing more and more tense. Only the most loyal, law-abiding Combines are allowed out on press day, and all week he's been anxiously checking for updates on the requirements. His superiors have him on a short lead, and there's no room for error. The rules are clear: one wrong move, and you'll face the consequences.

Yesterday, all Combines who still have the privilege of venturing beyond their apartments were gathered in the theatre. Representatives from Head Office stood on the stage and told us of the wonderful opportunity and privilege bestowed upon us. We listened, our face burning with the injustice of it all. *Our friend is dead due to their negligence, and we're supposed to be grateful?*

'This is the first time the outside world will be gaining access to a Combine community,' the woman addressing us began. Her voluminous blonde hair was parted in the centre, and she held the microphone with fingers covered in diamond rings. She strode across the stage, perfectly balanced in her stiletto heels. 'It is the first time newly merged Combines, still undergoing rehabilitation, will be shown to the world. Never before have The Village's residents been considered ready for public eyes. You are the exception. You, your faces, your stories, will go down in history.'

We sat beside Noah-Lucas, who kept nudging us with their elbow. 'Can you believe this?' they whispered excitedly. 'They're letting the outside world in. Ellie will be able to see what it's like for us in here.'

We forced ourselves to smile and nod, resisting the urge to shake them.

The ease with which Noah-Lucas has moved on from Lara-Jay's death hurts. We've seen them every day since the lockdown was lifted, and each day they dismiss our concerns. 'I think Nathan's right, Laurie-Amelia. I think you need to start trusting the Support Workers more. Otherwise you'll never be at peace.'

Despite our best efforts to get through to them, to encourage them to think critically and question what they hear, they remain all too willing to accept what they're told and do as they're asked. *We mustn't judge them, Amelia. They've such little life experience. Too young, it seems, to have anything but faith in authority.*

Still, it's so difficult to listen to them. Most of the time, Noah-Lucas just regurgitates the lines Callie's fed them. We know because they're Nathan's lines, too.

Usually, we go to the library, and Noah-Lucas lets us cry quietly into their soft, pale neck as they read. We wait until Nathan and Callie are far enough away, browsing the shelves, before we whisper urgently, 'If Combine are allowing vulnerable people to merge, then they need to make sure they're providing the proper support and resources for them. They had a duty of care to Lara and Jay. And they failed them. *They killed them.*'

No matter how we word it, Noah-Lucas disagrees. 'Lara lied, Laurie-Amelia,' he always says. 'She deceived them. She deceived us all. How could they have known Lara and Jay weren't a match when she was such a good liar?'

We didn't share Noah-Lucas's enthusiasm for the speeches from Head Office. We listened closely, hoping for a mention of Lara-Jay or a moment of silence in their honour. But the acknowledgement never came.

As the event went on, everyone around us seemed to become captivated by the speakers. 'Come Thursday,' they announced, 'The Village will open its doors to the world. Seize this opportunity bestowed upon you. Show the public the transformative power of merging. Showcase the joy and harmony that defines our community. Pave the way for progress and prosperity.'

The lights dimmed, and the room erupted with cheers and applause. Nathan's eyes were on us, so we joined in, our throat and hands aching from the intensity of our feigned enthusiasm. As we made our way back to our apartment, away from the pulsating beats of the music and the excited chatter of Combines gathered in tight groups, unease settled over us. 'Is everything okay, Laurie-Amelia?' Nathan asked. 'You've gone awfully pale.'

'I'm fine,' we said, forcing a smile. 'Just exhausted from all the excitement.'

We spent the night going over everything that had happened. Our medication being altered made it difficult to focus, and we had to fight sleep as the day's final dose kicked in. *Head Office wants us to believe this is an opportunity to showcase the Merge, to show the world how wonderful life is here. But that's not why they're coming, is it? No. It's Lara-Jay's death that has drawn them.*

We sat up in bed, refusing to let the fatigue win, our eyes heavy but our heart racing. *Yes. They're coming to investigate Lara-Jay's suicide, to find out what went wrong. You know what they're going to do, don't you? They'll paint Lara as a good-for-nothing junkie. A liar. They'll use the visit as an opportunity to destroy her reputation once and for all.*

We nodded. It was suddenly so obvious. Combine thinks if they put on a big enough show, we'll forget; we'll accept their narrative that Lara was an untrustworthy addict who deceived them. That it was *her* fault this happened, *her* fault she died, not theirs.

Another realisation hit. Yes, some journalists are eager for the glossy inside scoop, happy to be shown the facilities and the supposed serenity of life here. But there will be others, too, reporters with different intentions. The ones driven to expose the hidden dangers lurking beneath the surface of the experiment.

And we'll help them, won't we, Mum?

Of course we will.

Gilded by the low afternoon sun, the courtyard is beautiful. The polished fountain hurts our eyes when we look at it, the water flowing like lava. There are more flowers than we remember, plant pots exploding with brilliant reds, purples, whites and pinks. We walk through the arches of purple hyssop, plump white roses and glossy laurel leaves. Although we've been to the courtyard many times, we can't remember this walkway. We try not to let the panic surface, pushing aside the prickling in our legs that comes each time a memory fades.

The arches are the same as those used in Commitment Ceremonies. *Have you had any luck remembering ours? Sometimes I think I glimpse a fragment of memory but then it slips away.* We look at the flowers, trying desperately to recall the time we spent beneath them, dressed in purple gowns, our faces covered by gauzy veils. But there's nothing. Not even a whisper.

A desk has been set up in front of the fountain, close enough that its glass surface is beaded with droplets carried by the breeze. Three suited women sit behind it, laptops open in front of them. One looks at us but doesn't smile. Beyond the fountain is the throng of reporters, camera crews and photographers. There's a fusillade of flashes and loud laughter. We go up on tiptoes, trying to see what's happening. 'Be patient, Laurie-Amelia,' Nathan says quietly. 'We'll join them shortly.'

The suited women stand. They lower their eyes, their chins tucked to their chests, as they thank us for our sacrifice. We nod and mutter a thank you. 'Ms Singh is due to be interviewed next,' one of the women tells Nathan. She looks in the direction of the crowd. 'It seems to be going really well. It was a little tense for a while – a few of the reporters were rather hard on the founders, and Mr Brightwell had quite a bit to answer for. But Noah-Lucas has won them over. They're such an exemplary Combine.'

We look at Nathan. 'Noah-Lucas?'

Nathan nods. 'They wanted to share their story. I didn't tell you because I didn't want you to feel pressured into going in front of the cameras. Laurie-Amelia, wait—'

But we're already walking away. We hurry round the fountain, weaving through the cameras and clusters of journalists, ignoring the bitter and sarcastic comments from the reporters we brush past.

We slow to a halt.

Noah-Lucas is sitting beside a woman we recognise. *Doesn't she usually interview celebrities? On that panel show? It is her, isn't it?* Noah-Lucas's hair, freshly cut, is slicked back. Their suit is green velvet, the collar a few shades darker than the rest of the jacket. On their pocket is the mandala stitched in gold thread. They're smiling, looking completely at ease in the spotlight. We remember Lucas talking about how Noah would change their look once they merged, and how excited he was to be stylish and confident.

The woman's hand rests gently on Noah-Lucas's arm as they tell her about their first bike ride since merging. We watch as they comically re-enact their cycling experience, miming steering through obstacles and dodging pedestrians. All the while, the woman's hand remains glued to their arm. *Is it to rein them in if their performance gets too over-the-top? Or stop them if they say something they shouldn't?*

Around us, the reporters watch, their faces lit up with amusement. Some lean forward, hanging on every word, microphones bristling. 'My mind feels clear and focused,' Noah-Lucas says. 'It's like I'm finally living in alignment with my true self. It's incredibly liberating. I wouldn't say there's any conflict at all. Just harmony.'

As the interview draws to a close, Noah-Lucas looks directly into the camera. They pause, compose themselves. We lick our lips, silently urging them to do the right thing, to mention Lara-Jay, to use this moment to ensure they're not forgotten. To clear Lara's name.

'Cancer once threatened to tear me apart,' they say, their voice loud and resolute. 'Cancer threatened to end my life. If it weren't for the Merge, I'd be dead. And here I am, stronger than I've ever been. I stand tall and proud as a survivor.' They smile. 'I owe my life to Combine.'

All around us, reporters applaud as though they've witnessed a miracle. But all we see are the lives Combine has lost. Lara-Jay plummeting from the bell tower. Father and daughter, trapped, forced to take their own lives.

Nausea rises in us as we push our way through the crowd. Noah-Lucas can't see what's happening. They're blind to the truth, willingly advocating for an experiment that has taken the lives of our friends.

We need Albie. Or Mary. Someone who loves us. Someone who would listen and believe our concerns. They need to know that Lara was a good person, that this narrative Combine is spreading, about her being a liar, a good-for-nothing junkie, is false. If Albie were here, we could tell him, and he could spread the word, take the truth beyond The Village.

We reach an empty bench and sit, leaning forward, putting our head between our legs, fighting for breath.

'I'm sorry I didn't tell you.'

We look up. Nathan's standing in front of us, his hands in his trouser pockets. 'Noah-Lucas wanted to put the tragedy of Lara-Jay's death into perspective by sharing their success story. May I?' He gestures at the bench. We nod, and he sits. For a moment, he just watches us in silence.

'Eliza's going to be making some big announcements in her interview, Laurie-Amelia. They're good things. Great things. But they're things I'd rather you heard from me.' He pauses, leaning closer. 'I'm under strict instruction not to divulge this information before Eliza, but like I keep saying, I trust you.' He holds our gaze, and we feel an urge to punch him. 'Look, Laurie-Amelia, Eliza's going to announce your trial as a major success. Merges for Participants with Alzheimer's will officially open to the public next month.' He smiles. 'Because of you, Laurie-Amelia, merging is going to be prescribed to treat Alzheimer's. No one will ever have to endure this disease again. All thanks to you.'

We stare at him. 'What? I'm being signed off? I can go home, back to Albie?'

'Not just yet. You'll be back with Albie soon, though, Laurie-Amelia. I promise. Your Merge isn't quite complete. They just—'

'The Merge is being opened to Alzheimer's patients, prescribed as a cure, even though I'm not finished yet?'

Nathan nods.

'But we don't know that the Alzheimer's didn't transfer. I still forget things. There are so many gaps in my memory, like the days before and after I merged. I still have no clue what happened. You said the memories would come back, but they haven't. And these arches.' We gesture at the walkway. 'I have no memory of them being here.'

'They're new, Laurie-Amelia. The courtyard has been specially decorated for today. And as for the gaps, blanks are normal. They just take time to return, that's all. You haven't forgotten anything. Not for weeks.'

That's not right, is it? We've hardly been able to think for ourselves. We've been so drugged up, I can't— 'Weeks? That's not... I don't think that's accurate, Nathan.'

He places his hand gently on our knee. 'You should be so proud of yourself, Laurie-Amelia. You've achieved what you set out to do, and you've done it in record time.' He gives our knee a small squeeze before moving his hand away. 'Please, don't overthink it. Combine knows what they're doing. You're free of Alzheimer's. All you've got to do is believe it, and you'll be back to your life sooner than you know it. Now, let's go and support Eliza, shall we?'

A hush replaces the low murmur as Eliza takes her seat beside the same woman who interviewed Noah-Lucas. Eliza's hair, usually neatly braided, is stuffed into a lopsided bun, and her makeup somehow contrives to make her look pale and ill. We look at the interviewer, so glamorous by comparison. *I know her name. I'm certain I do. We'd be able to remember if it weren't for the Alzheimer's. That's evidence, isn't it? Proof we're not cured?*

We could tell Nathan, right here in front of the journalists, that we can't remember the woman's name, that we're still forgetting. It would make headlines worldwide. We wonder how Combine would spin our story. They couldn't use Alzheimer's as an excuse, like they used Lara's addiction. They'd have to fabricate a different narrative, perhaps pin our forgetting on our grief, and in doing so, shift the blame back onto Lara.

We think of our windowless bedroom, the endless hours trapped inside, the Combines confined to their apartments, watching the world pass by. We think of Albie, and the prospect of going home – perhaps even our real home, the fairytale cottage we had to surrender to the Combines. We can't risk saying anything.

The journalist beside us clears her throat. When we first sat down, she was so excited by our arrival that she stood and curtseyed as she thanked us for our sacrifice. 'Jennifer Ferguson,' she said, both of her hands warmly clasping ours. 'From Sky News.' Her smile widened, revealing a slight gap between her front teeth, something oddly familiar that tugged at the edges of our memory. 'It's such a pleasure to meet you, Laurie-Amelia. What's it been like for you here? Has everything gone as well as you'd hoped?'

We started to respond, but Nathan interjected. 'You have been explicitly told not to question Combines. Utter another word to Laurie-Amelia, and I'll see you escorted off site.'

Jennifer flushed, apologised and slid back into her seat without so much as a glance in our direction.

Eliza stands. The silence intensifies, stretching taut. The reporters are hungry. Noah-Lucas was merely the appetiser; this is what they're really here for. Something sensational.

Eliza steps towards the camera, catching our eye. Nathan nods and gives her a quick thumbs-up. We don't smile. Eliza is about to announce our trial a success and she's said nothing, asked nothing, not bothered to check if we're okay, if we're still encountering blanks with our memory.

Nathan bites his lip, his fingers drumming a nervous rhythm on his thigh. Is he anxious for Eliza's sake, or his own? Perhaps it's not nerves but excitement. Declaring the Alzheimer's trial a success not only removes heat from Lara-Jay's suicide. It makes him a hero.

'Hello everyone.' Eliza's voice is surprisingly calm. Someone must have prepared her, trained her for this moment. The world is watching. Her delivery needs to be flawless. 'My name is Eliza Singh. I was the Support Worker responsible for Lara-Jay, who tragically passed away ten days ago.' *Ten days? Is that really all it's been?* 'As their Support Worker, I had the privilege of walking alongside Lara-Jay on their journey. I knew them both as Jay and Lara, father and daughter, and as Lara-Jay, the Combine who sought to cure their addiction.'

She pauses. Swallows. 'Lara-Jay's absence leaves a void in my heart, and in the hearts of all those who knew and loved them.' Another pause. Longer, this time. Long enough for us to see reporters exchanging curious looks. 'When such a tragedy occurs, it is natural to seek answers and to assign blame. I understand the scrutiny surrounding my role as Lara-Jay's Support Worker, but I urge you all to recognise that mental health challenges are complex and multifaceted. While I bear the weight of responsibility as their Support Worker, I also acknowledge that suicide is a deeply personal and often well-hidden struggle. Despite my very best efforts to provide support, Lara-Jay's decision was ultimately beyond my control.'

She takes another step forward. 'Allow me to shed a little light on the reality that our world faces today. As the climate crisis escalates, recent data reveals a troubling rise in suicide and mental health issues, particularly among the younger generations. Here in the United Kingdom, we have forged a path that allows us to move forward with renewed hope and genuine optimism. The Merge offers a lifeline for those who might otherwise succumb to that dangerous, endemic hopelessness from which large – swathes – of the planet are currently suffering. Through the Merge, we can unite in a profound act of solidarity, sharing a common purpose, and create countless brighter tomorrows. By embracing the Merge, we honour the memory of our beloved Lara-Jay and ensure that their death was not in vain. Let us pave the way for a future where hope prevails, and the precious bonds of humanity endure. Thank you.'

Eliza takes a deep breath, nods and resumes her seat. Feeling Nathan's eyes on us, we join in with the gentle applause.

'Thank you, Eliza,' the interviewer says with a smile. 'We will now invite questions from the audience.'

There's no doubt in our mind that the question-and-answer session has been rehearsed. The woman hosting the discussion carefully selects reporters, repeatedly returning to the same few, seemingly blind to the other raised hands. When the questions come, Eliza doesn't hesitate, doesn't miss a beat. Every answer is seamlessly delivered, each one painting Combine in the same flattering light.

A reporter towards the front, who has already asked two questions, is offered the opportunity for a third. 'Do you have any updates on the other Experimental Participants?'

Eliza nods. 'As you know, Noah-Lucas is thriving and perfectly healthy. You saw for yourselves how phenomenally well they are doing as a Combine. They're now enjoying the carefree and fulfilling life every teenager deserves to experience, free from the burden of disease. As for Laurie-Amelia, their journey has also been nothing short of remarkable.'

'Smile,' Nathan whispers.

Then the camera is on us, and Eliza's talking about the *remarkable reversal* of our symptoms, how *no trace of dementia remains*. We want to shake our head, to correct her, to tell the cameras and the crowd that there are still blanks – so many gaps we can't fill. But Nathan's hand rests firmly on our arm, a silent warning. We know we can't. If we ever want to get out of The Village, we need to comply.

So we do as we're told and smile.

The reporter sitting beside us can't help herself. 'Congratulations, Laurie-Amelia,' she whispers. 'I'm delighted for you.'

Eliza stands and clears her throat. A camera is pointed directly at us.

'In light of the success of our Experimental Trials,' she begins, 'it brings me the greatest pleasure to announce that Merges for Participants with terminal illnesses, including Alzheimer's, will be available to the public as early as next month.'

The audience grows loud in their excitement. Questions are called out over one another. *Is this the end of terminal illness? Are you saying that Combine have discovered a cure for cancer? What will this mean for people already in the late stages of Alzheimer's?* But they're ignored. Eliza listens only to the reporter at the front. 'And Benjamin-Annie?' he asks. 'How are they?'

We straighten in our seat.

Nathan tenses beside us.

Eliza looks directly at the camera, just as Noah-Lucas did when they made their closing statement. She smiles so convincingly that it seems genuine. 'I am delighted,' she announces, her voice ringing with pride, 'to share that, last week, Benjamin-Annie gave birth to a perfectly healthy baby boy.'

We don't have time for the news to sink in. Confusion clouds us as we frown and turn to the reporter beside us. 'What did she just—' But Nathan pulls us to our feet. He escorts us quickly through the swelling crowd of reporters shouting questions over one another, demanding to be heard.

'Come on, Laurie-Amelia.' Nathan's grip tightens as he rushes us past the desk manned by the three women. They stand, craning their necks. 'What's going on?' one asks as we pass. 'What's caused all the commotion?' Nathan's hand is tight on our wrist as he drags us away, back through the arches. He walks so fast we have to jog to keep up. 'Benjamin-Annie has had their baby? They've given birth? Is that what Eliza just said?'

That can't be right, can it? Am I getting confused?

Nathan quickens his pace. We stumble along, our mind racing. That's definitely what Eliza said. We're certain of it. Benjamin-Annie has given birth to a perfectly healthy baby boy. We try to pull away from Nathan, but his grip is too tight. His fingers coil round our wrist. 'What's going on?' we say. 'You're scaring me.'

'There's nothing to be scared of, Laurie-Amelia. I just need to get you home.'

Only once we're inside our apartment, with the door locked and the world silent, do we realise what's just happened: Nathan dragged us away before we could hear any details, before we could find out how Benjamin-Annie is, how they're coping since giving birth.

Since giving birth. They've given birth. They've...

We falter, stepping back. There was no mention of their health. No confirmation that they even survived.

Nathan leans against the door, his chest rising and falling in deep, irregular breaths. All this time, he's kept us away from Benjamin-Annie and their baby. 'I trust you,' he always says. But he doesn't.

'You lied to me, Nathan. Repeatedly. Why didn't you tell me about Benjamin-Annie's baby?'

His breathing steadies, his chest no longer heaving. 'I didn't lie. I kept the truth hidden. That's not the same thing.'

'When did they give birth?'

Nathan looks at the floor. 'The day of your Passing,' he says quietly.

It takes a moment for the words to sink in. Tears brim and then spill.

'Laurie-Amelia...'

We shake our head. It can't be right. Benjamin-Annie couldn't have given birth the same day we Passed... the same day Lara-Jay killed themselves. Nathan wouldn't have kept this from us for so long. We look at him, his flushed face blurred by our tears. 'You said you'd tell me as soon as there was something to tell.'

'It's not as though you were in any state to visit them. You could hardly get out of bed, Laurie-Amelia.'

'I didn't *know*!' we shout. 'You didn't tell me. If I'd known, I'd have pulled myself together. I'd have done everything I could to be there for them. You know I would have.'

We recall the days that followed Lara-Jay's death, when we couldn't get out of bed, our grief a heavy blanket we couldn't shake. Would we really have been able to visit Benjamin-Annie, knowing they had just given birth and were so vulnerable? Could we have summoned the strength to lift ourselves out of that deep, dark pit if we'd known?

Nathan presses his palms against his lips, his eyes betraying his struggle to stay composed. 'They needed the time alone. Visiting them would have been inappropriate. They're a new parent, Laurie-Amelia. And a new Combine. There's so much for them to adjust to. They need the time alone. They need to bond with Teddy.'

We wipe our cheeks dry with our sleeve. 'Teddy?'

'Teddy Benjamin Miller,' Nathan says softly. 'He's a beautiful little boy.'

We move into the lounge, needing to sit, to steady ourselves. We sink into the sofa, resting our head in our hands. We think of Teddy, Ben and Annie. We imagine the love they must feel, tangled with an overwhelming anxiety, knowing the weight Teddy will carry growing up in a world that judges before it understands.

Nathan has visited them. He has seen Benjamin-Annie as a parent. He has met Teddy, likely held him, maybe even given him a small gift. And he hasn't mentioned a word of it to us. All those times we asked after Benjamin-Annie, he grew angry, accusing us of being interrogative. We think of him coming through the door, always smiling, always acting chipper, even when he clearly wasn't in a good mood. Not once did we question where he had been.

Nathan has followed us into the lounge. He stands by the window, looking out at the complex, where reporters are still gathered in the courtyard. They'll be hearing all about Benjamin-Annie and their new baby, learning everything we're desperate to know.

Resentment and hatred flood through us.

But then we steel ourselves. *Why should we believe anything Eliza's reporting? Or anything Nathan tells us? Think about it, Mum. They've already lied to the media about us being cured of Alzheimer's. They could be lying about this, too. For all we know, there is no baby.*

'I need to see them,' we say.

Nathan turns away from the window. He tugs gently at his

cheeks, stretching his lower eyelids downward to reveal the raw, reddened skin beneath. 'Laurie-Amelia...'

'You're still not going to let me, are you?'

'Not yet. But soon.'

We go to argue but stop ourselves. Angering him won't do us any favours, though part of us is too furious to care. Our mouth opens, then closes. *No. Don't. He holds the key to our freedom, remember.*

'You need to stop them from opening the Merge to people with Alzheimer's,' we say instead. 'They can't tell the world I'm cured, that others with Alzheimer's will be cured if they sign up. It's a lie. I'm not cured. I don't *feel* cured.'

'Why won't you believe in yourself, Laurie-Amelia? Why are you refusing to recognise the astonishing progress you've made?'

'I still forget things... The blanks—'

Our watch beeps. So does Nathan's. 'You're cured, Laurie-Amelia,' he says, silencing his watch. 'You're free of Alzheimer's. I just wish you'd enjoy it.' He retreats to the kitchen to prepare our pills.

We stand and move to the window, staring out at the reporters in the courtyard. We imagine all the others doing the same, those Combines we saw earlier, rows of ghostly faces peering from their windows. We look at the ceiling, wondering who might be just above us. We imagine them, this featureless figure, observing the outside world from their lounge, just as we are.

When we wake from our nap, Eliza is here.

'She's staying with you while I have my interview,' Nathan says. 'I don't want you being alone, and I think you've had enough of the press for one day.' He pauses, glancing towards the lounge, his voice dropping. 'She wants to talk. Hear her out, Laurie-Amelia.' He squeezes our shoulder gently before leaving the apartment.

We remain where we are, taking a moment to compose ourselves before entering the lounge. We like Eliza. She has always listened to our concerns, always taken the time to understand our worries. It's why we wanted her as our Support Worker, why her announcement of our 'cure' feels like such a betrayal.

She's sitting on the sofa and stands as we enter, awkwardly tugging her sleeves down over her hands. 'I'm so sorry,' she says. 'We were under strict instruction not to mention Benjamin-Annie's baby. They said it would send you and Noah-Lucas spiralling to hear such news in the depths of your grief. You had to process Lara-Jay's death first. I wasn't allowed to mention it. Not until today's interview.'

We move towards the partially completed puzzle laid out on the carpet. It's five hundred pieces, a step up from the last. The image it will eventually create is of a colourful, striped hot-air balloon. 'Want to help me with this?' we ask.

Eliza remains where she is, watching as we sit cross-legged in front of the puzzle and begin sifting through the pile of red pieces. 'I wanted to tell you. Really, Laurie-Amelia, I did.'

'I know,' we say, focusing on the pieces in front of us. 'I understand.'

She moves closer, kneeling beside us. 'The last thing I wanted to do was cause you more upset. But I had to follow orders.'

We pick up a piece and test it. It doesn't fit. 'I understand, Eliza. You couldn't tell me the news while I was grieving. I get it.'

She watches as we press a red jigsaw piece into its place.

We look at her. 'Please stop worrying. I'm fine. Honestly.'

We're convincing, we think. We're well versed in ridding people of their guilty consciences. *Of course you only get so cross with my mother because you love her so much. Of course you didn't mean to hurt her. Of course you only hit her because you care.*

We work on the puzzle in silence. Eliza keeps watching, keeps apologising. 'Do you blame me?' she says eventually. 'Do you think it's my fault Lara-Jay…'

We keep our eyes on the puzzle, carefully placing a yellow piece.

'I thought I could save them,' she says quietly. 'I thought, if I took them on myself – cared for them – that I'd get them through. Jay was so mentally strong. I thought he'd… overpower… Lara. He should have… I should have double-checked their compatibility scores. I should have tested her again. They never seemed compatible, did they? I don't know why I didn't question it.' She wipes her eyes quickly. 'I'm so sorry, Laurie-Amelia. For all of it.'

We continue working on the puzzle, and she continues to watch.

'Is there anything I can do to make it up to you?'

We pause, our hand hovering over a piece, an idea forming.

'Take me to Lara-Jay's apartment.'

She remains silent as we sift through the orange pieces, testing one that doesn't fit. Then, finally, 'You know Nathan won't allow it.'

We look up at her and smile. 'He doesn't need to know. Isn't that what we've just been talking about? How sometimes you have to keep things from people… to protect them?'

She hesitates. 'It would really help you to visit?'

We nod. 'I need it, Eliza. I need the closure.'

Before we can enter Lara-Jay's apartment, Eliza insists that we put on gloves and protect our shoes with plastic covers made from carrier bags. 'There can't be any sign of us having been here,' she says when we ask if it's really necessary. 'If Nathan finds out I've let you in, he'll be furious. We can't stay long.'

We stand outside the door. Apartment 86. The number etched into the small brass plate. Taking a deep breath, we steady ourselves. We know what we're here for: to see Lara-Jay as they really were, not the version Combine is trying to force on us. We want to see how they lived, to understand them better, see Village life through their eyes. We want to know what they were going through, what made it all unbearable. But it feels intrusive suddenly, to be entering their apartment without their permission. Like a terrible invasion of their privacy.

'Come on then.' Eliza's holding the door open, waiting for us to step inside.

We move slowly through the doorway, imagining we are Lara-Jay returning home from a walk or a class, and this is what we see.

The hallway is identical to ours. The same minimalist decor. The same hardwood floors. The same neutral colour scheme. We look around for signs of life: a pair of shoes, a coat, a set of keys. But there's nothing. Everything is tidied away. It's how the Support Workers insist we keep our apartments, but we never imagined Lara-Jay conforming. We pictured them refusing to make their bed, refusing to wipe down surfaces or dust the windowsills.

We'd hoped, we realise, for signs of resistance.

'Has the apartment been cleaned?' we ask. 'Or is this how Lara-Jay left it?'

'It hasn't been touched,' Eliza says.

Of course it hasn't. They haven't bothered to properly investigate what happened to Lara-Jay. They're too busy appeasing the press.

We step into the lounge. Disappointment washes over us. The sofa and footstool are the colour of oatmeal. The carpet is cream. A partially completed puzzle lies on the coffee table. We recognise the pink and white pattern; it's the same puzzle we finished months ago, the one Noah-Lucas helped us with.

How will we understand Lara-Jay's anguish – how will we make sense of what they confided in us – if their experience was no different from ours?

'Are you okay, Laurie-Amelia?'

We look at the puzzle, at the small patch of pink pieces forming a segment of the sky. *Could that have been it, do you think? The difference between us? We had help. Company. Noah-Lucas was always stopping by. Why didn't we ever do the same for Lara-Jay?*

It was the silence, we know. But realising it now feels futile – so hollow, so painfully selfish.

'Not too close, Laurie-Amelia,' Eliza whispers when we near the window. 'We can't have you being spotted.'

This, at least, is different. Lara-Jay's view wasn't of the courtyard and the expanse of grass leading towards the library, but of the sports complex and the tennis courts. *Could that have made a difference? Could they have seen something that pushed them over the edge?* We know we're grasping at straws. If anything, their view was better than ours. We would have liked to watch the tennis matches during our time trapped inside.

A doubles match is in progress. We watch a Support Worker ace a Combine.

'Hurry along, Laurie-Amelia,' Eliza whispers. 'We need to go soon.'

She lingers awkwardly in the lounge, keeping close to the wall as we move into the kitchen. The white pearl countertops are clear and clean, the cupboards closed. The tea towels hanging from the oven door look untouched, their folds crisp and neat, as if freshly pressed. We glance behind us before opening a cupboard. We're not supposed to touch.

Tins of peaches and packets of noodles are lined up in neat rows. There's a half-eaten chocolate bar tucked in the corner, bearing the impression of teeth.

Eliza coughs in the other room. We jump and quickly shut the cupboard. The door bangs shut. We leave the kitchen and pass back through the lounge. Eliza stands just where we left her, smiling tightly.

We make for the bedroom and pause in the doorway, staring at the lived-in room. So unlike the rest of the apartment.

Here it is. What we came for. The real them.

The bed is unmade, the duvet fashioned into a deep nest, pillows tossed randomly, some cases half off. Clothes are strewn across the floor, shoes abandoned haphazardly, the pairs separated. *This is where they existed, where they must have spent most of their time.* The thought makes us uncomfortable. Like ours, their bedroom is windowless. We imagine them wasting away in bed, deprived of natural light, no distractions to quieten their hectic mind.

On the shelf above the bed, grinning teddy bears are lined up in neat rows. The larger bears at the back, the smaller ones at the front. Untouched, it seems, by the chaos surrounding them. Our chest tightens. How carefully the bears have been arranged. *Was it Lara looking after them, do you think? Or was it Jay, keeping them neat in some desperate attempt to hold on to his little girl?*

We step slowly into the room and place a gloved hand on the duvet, irrationally searching for a trace of warmth. 'Lara-Jay,' we whisper, the words catching in our throat, 'I'm so sorry.'

Their mirror is positioned exactly like ours, opposite the bed. We imagine them waking here, confronted by their own reflection, Lara's cry, sharp and raw, the first time she woke and saw her dad looking back at her. *She threw up at the thought of it. Can you imagine how scared she must have been when it became her reality? No wonder she couldn't cope.*

On the bedside table lies an open notebook, a broken pencil resting on it. Behind the notebook is a framed photograph of Kath and the boys, Kath smiling brightly, sandwiched between her sons. We pick up the notebook, and the pencil falls to the floor. Most of the page is dark with heavy shading. The lead must have snapped under the pressure of their strokes.

We picture them, hunched over the notebook, manically colouring. We see the lead snap. And something inside of them breaking with it. *If the lead hadn't broken, if they'd been able to continue pouring their distress onto the page, would they still be here?* We turn to the next page. It's completely filled in – a solid block of grey. And the next. And the next. All the way to the end.

We check the door for Eliza before opening the bedside table. Inside, there's a stack of photographs. We flick through them. They're of Jay, Lara, Kath and the boys. In each photo, there's a hole punched clean through Jay's chest. Made, we imagine, with the pencil. We tuck a photo into our pocket and quickly return the rest to the drawer.

We notice a brown teddy bear tucked between the pillows and pick it up, turning it over in our hands, tracing its stitched smile, its bright plastic eyes. Its fur is well worn, matted from years of affection. It must have been their favourite, the cherished one. *Doesn't it remind you of Waddles? Remember how his wings became frayed from so much love?*

We bring the bear to our nose and inhale softly.

A shadow of grief settles over us.

Lara was still young enough to want her teddy, to bring it with her and find comfort in its presence. She was only a child. And she had no say in any of this.

We close our eyes.

She didn't want this. She never wanted this.

We allow ourselves to remember her, to truly remember. We don't push away the memories as we usually do. Even when they come flooding in, threatening to overwhelm us, we welcome them. We breathe deeply, inviting them in.

We're sitting with Lara at the table in The Oasis. Her hood is up, and she's sulking, pushing pasta around her plate with her fork. The scene shifts – now Jay is talking to us, his voice tight with desperation. He's at his wit's end. *This is our last hope, the only way to keep my daughter alive.* Then we're in the middle of a session, sitting in the circle in the white room. Lara is slumped in her chair, scowling as Jay speaks about her past, telling us how difficult it is to trust her as much as he wants to. *Even when she's popping to the shops*, he says, *I become unbearably anxious. Sometimes I follow her. And I feel terrible about it.*

The scene changes again, and Lara's smiling at us, comforting us because we've forgotten something. *It doesn't matter*, she's saying. *I'll remind you if you forget.* We're at Ben and Annie's apartment, and Lara's angry about something Jay's said. She's scowling, her arms tightly folded across her chest. *You know how I hid drugs from them for all those years? I stuffed them in the soft toys she bought me every birthday and Christmas. Fucking soft toys.*

Our eyes snap open.

We look down at the faded brown bear smiling up at us.

You don't think they... Our fingers trace the seam, hesitating. *No, they wouldn't have. They couldn't have.* A quick glance towards the door, and then, carefully, we begin to untie the stitching, parting the worn fabric. Our fingers slip inside, sifting through the soft stuffing.

Nothing. See? I told you they wouldn't have—

Then we feel it. Our breath catches. We dig deeper, our fingers brushing against something solid and foreign. Slowly, we pull out a small plastic bag filled with pills.

Fucking hell.

A pause, our heart racing.

Are these—

'Laurie-Amelia?'

We jump. The bag slips from our hand, hitting the floor, scattering a few of the pills across the oak boards. Little grey tablets, the kind we swallow every day, lie like tiny pebbles strewn across the wood. Eliza's eyes widen, her shock mirroring ours. 'What... Where did you get these?'

'It's... They were inside the bear.'

Eliza's gaze shifts between the pills and the bear in our hands.

We swallow hard, our heart pounding. 'It's their medication, isn't it?' Our eyes drift to the shelf of bears, their stitched smiles suddenly sinister.

Eliza approaches the bed, reaching up to the shelf. She pulls down a large white bear wearing a blue beret. Lifting the bear's dress, she finds the stitching undone underneath. We watch, holding our breath, as her hand disappears inside the bear.

'No,' she whispers. 'No. No. No.'

Then she's moving quickly, pulling bears from the shelf. A small pink bear with a red heart stitched on its front topples and falls to the floor with a soft thud. We stare, disbelieving, as Eliza pulls open the teddies one by one. Baggies full of pills spill out with the stuffing.

We use Eliza's phone to call Nathan, and he arrives quickly, his expression unreadable as he steps into the room. His eyes widen at the sight of Eliza, slumped on Lara-Jay's bed, sobbing inconsolably. Around her lie the eviscerated teddy bears, their stuffing and pills scattered across the floor.

We hurry over to Nathan, overcome with relief at the sight of him. 'We found Lara-Jay's medication,' we blurt, the words tumbling out in a rush. 'It was hidden inside their teddies.'

Nathan frowns, his brow creasing as he shakes his head. 'Wait, Laurie-Amelia, what are you talking about? Lara-Jay's medication? Hidden in teddies?'

'They weren't taking it, Nathan,' we say just as quickly. 'That's why they killed themselves. It's why they died. They must have been in agony. You're always saying the medication makes merging bearable. How could they possibly have aligned in so much pain?'

Nathan's expression hardens as he calls for help, and soon two men we don't recognise arrive to escort Eliza from the apartment. 'Can you believe it,' we ask once they've left. 'Can you believe we found—' But Nathan is furious – angrier than we've ever seen him. He turns to us, his voice cold and sharp. 'I don't care what you found, Laurie-Amelia. You lied to me. You tricked Eliza into bringing you here.'

'I didn't trick—'

'Don't,' he snaps. 'There's no way she'd have agreed to bring you if you hadn't done something manipulative.'

We stare, stunned by his reaction. We've uncovered the truth everyone was searching for, discovered why Lara-Jay's Merge went so catastrophically wrong, and now we're being *punished* for it.

'And if I hadn't come?' we shout. 'If I hadn't come, we'd still not know why Lara-Jay took their life, Nathan. It's not because Lara lied. It's because they were terrified – terrified of becoming addicted to these pills.'

Nathan grabs our shoulders, his fingers digging in. He shake us. 'How can I trust you, Laurie-Amelia?' His voice cracks, and suddenly we realise this isn't just anger. It's something deeper. He's hurt. 'How can I give you any freedom when, the few hours I leave you alone, this is what you do? Combines need to listen to their Support Workers. I know what's best. I keep you safe. If you begin lying to me...'

Tears well in his eyes. We've never seen him cry, not even when Lara-Jay died. A memory flashes – Tony gripping our shoulders as he wept, telling us how much he loved our mother. *Don't you see? They're all the same. Destined to hurt us.*

'I won't do it again,' we say quickly. 'I'm sorry, Nathan.'

His grip loosens immediately, his hands falling away. 'You've done well, Laurie-Amelia,' he says quietly. 'What you've uncovered, it's – great. Vital.' He looks at us, his eyes still glistening, the anger in them fading. 'I just wish you'd been honest with me. I wish we'd discovered it together.'

We walk with Noah-Lucas. They're quieter than usual but insist they're okay. 'It's just been a lot, hasn't it? These past few days. They've completely wiped me out.'

We study them closely. They've been so full of energy, so healthy, we've never seen them drained like this. Like Noah was. Our alarmed expression makes them laugh. 'I'm not sick, Laurie-Amelia,' they say. 'I'm just tired. It's been pretty emotional. First losing Lara-Jay, then the news about Benjamin-Annie, and now finding out Lara-Jay was never taking their tablets. It's a lot to process.'

We nod, understanding their feelings all too well. The regular announcements don't help. You can never go too long without a reminder of Lara-Jay's suicide. *Your health is our priority. Stay on the path to alignment success and always take your medication as prescribed.*

For us, how we're feeling varies from day to day, hour to hour. The shock comes in waves. There are moments when we feel level-headed and logical: Lara-Jay wasn't taking their medication, so they couldn't align; this drove them to madness, and they took their own life. How could we have known they weren't swallowing their pills when even Eliza didn't realise what was going on? How could we possibly have saved them?

At other times, we are tortured by guilt. If we'd gone to their apartment, if we'd made the effort to visit, we'd have seen the bears. The memory would have surfaced, and we'd have investigated. We'd have found the pills and saved them. Lara would have been able to communicate. They'd have merged properly. They'd be clean, and they'd be happy. They'd be alive.

A Combine passes us on their bike, ringing their bell. Noah-Lucas gives a half-hearted wave. 'Have you asked Callie if you can visit Benjamin-Annie?' we ask.

They nod. 'She says they're not ready for visitors. They've still not progressed beyond their accommodation. Something to do with their mobility. They want to make sure everyone's safe. I mean, with the way things are, they can't be too careful.'

We look behind us. Callie and Nathan are talking, distracted.

'Lara-Jay died, Noah-Lucas,' we say, our voice low. 'They died because of the Merge. They didn't keep them safe.'

Noah-Lucas sighs. 'How many times can we have this conversation, Laurie-Amelia? They died because they weren't compatible, and because they lied about taking their medication. Combine did everything they could. *Eliza* did everything she could. Everyone tried to keep them safe.' They shake their head. 'You can't continue to blame everyone for their death. It won't bring them back. It'll only make you miserable.'

Nathan and Callie catch up with us, and we don't say anything else. We walk in silence as Noah-Lucas tells us about their cooking class. They've learned to make soufflé.

Are they for real? Do they really see nothing wrong with the way Lara-Jay was treated?

No response comes.

Mum?

Eventually, a reply. Faint and distant, but there. *They're sweet boys.*

Naïve, you mean.

We're still in bed when Nathan arrives to take us to art therapy. He makes us a strong coffee. 'The morning announcements must have finished an hour ago,' he says, handing us the mug. 'Are you sure you're feeling okay? Your sleep score is terrible.'

We nod, bringing the mug to our lips. The smell hits, a nauseating reminder of why we usually avoid coffee. But we're exhausted, so we take a sip, wincing as we swallow. Burnt charcoal. How we ever drank coffee for pleasure, we're unsure. 'I'm fine,' we say. 'Just tired. This week has been really full on.'

The truth is, we've hardly slept. Our supposed success as a Combine means we're being weaned off the drugs that have cocooned us so far. On the lower dosage, our dreams don't fully form, which is a blessing, but the bad thoughts are still there. Last night, we kept jolting awake, convinced that someone was in the room with us. We turned on the light each time, checking under the bed and in the wardrobe for whoever had just spoken.

'It's certainly been a busy few days,' Nathan agrees. He sits on the end of our bed. A faint creak escapes the frame as he settles. 'You'll have to make sure you nap later, or else you'll find today a struggle.'

The mattress dips slightly as he adjusts his position, turning to face us. 'I've been reflecting on what you did for Lara-Jay. I know you were seeking catharsis through understanding their perspective. But you were also seeking justice in a way, weren't you? You wanted to clear their name.'

We take another sip. So bitter. Like medicine.

'You've ensured that Lara-Jay's memory isn't tarnished by misconceptions, and you've provided closure for all those who loved them. I'm not saying you went about it in the right way – you didn't – but your intentions were good.

You wanted to honour their memory by understanding their pain, and you've done that. You're a remarkably good friend, Laurie-Amelia. And, well, I feel you deserve the opportunity to be a good friend to Benjamin-Annie.'

A smile tugs at our lips, but we don't allow it to fully form. We lift the mug, letting its rim shield the faint curve of our mouth. Nathan's words are so often cryptic. We mustn't get excited. Not until what he's telling us is clear. We fight to keep our voice level. 'You mean I can see them?'

Nathan nods, and we lower the mug, unable to suppress the smile.

We must look ridiculous, grinning like this. But the relief is overwhelming; our worst fears can't possibly be true. If we're being taken to see them, then Benjamin-Annie must be alive. They must be okay.

'We'll head over there this afternoon. I've spoken with Angela. She said Benjamin-Annie is thrilled that you'll be visiting.' Nathan chuckles at our delight. 'I have even more good news for you. You're being signed off, Laurie-Amelia. In a matter of weeks, you'll be out of The Village and restarting your real life.'

'I'm... What? I'm going home? To Albie?'

He nods. 'Combine is hosting a farewell party – a big event – at Alexandra Palace next week. They want to celebrate you, Laurie-Amelia, to give you the recognition you deserve.'

Warmth spreads through our chest. We're going *home*. We're getting out of here, back to Albie, leaving all this behind. 'I can't believe it,' we say. 'You're serious?'

'Completely.'

Our smile fades, our mind flickering back to last night – the frantic checks, the shaking hands as we scanned our empty room, only calming down because we knew Nathan would be there to check on us in the morning. Without him... without the Support Workers...

How will we cope?

A tightness grips our chest. 'Nathan, I don't think I'm ready. I can barely cope here on the reduced medication. How will I manage outside?'

His expression softens. 'You won't be on your own. You'll be living in Combine housing and receiving twenty-four seven care. You'll be monitored just like in The Village. It's crucial you move forward, Laurie-Amelia, to showcase your progress to the world.' He pats our leg under the duvet. 'I'll leave you to finish your coffee in peace. I'll be in the kitchen making breakfast if you need me.'

We don't finish the coffee. We get out of bed and hurry to the bathroom. In the shower, uncontrollable laughter bursts from us. As we dry and dress, we giggle, overcome with relief. We're getting out of here.

We walk with Nathan, holding tightly to the string of a cloud-shaped balloon. It floats above us, declaring *So Happy!* The air is crisp, but the sun shines brightly, and the sky is a perfect, uninterrupted blue. Nathan guides us towards the tree-lined path that leads to the theatre. Our balloon bobs as we walk, eager to escape and float away.

What do you think Teddy will look like? Do you think we'll be able to recognise Ben in his features? You do remember Ben, don't you?

No response.

We think of Ben, and his image forms clearly in our mind: his kind eyes, his short curls, his studded nose. A beautiful man inside and out. How delighted Annie would be if he was mirrored in their son.

We turn down a narrow path we don't remember seeing before. A short wooden sign driven into the grass reads *PRIVATE*. 'It's okay,' Nathan says. 'We have permission. The sign's there to discourage intrusion. You'll soon see why. We are on our way to The Enclave, home to the youngest residents in The Village.'

The Enclave is a part of The Village rarely referred to by the Support Workers, and only when they think we're not listening. We're not sure why they bother with the secrecy; everyone knows it exists.

Teachers can be that way. Unnecessarily secretive. We once worked with a woman who kept her class timetable hidden so that the poor children never knew what to expect. It made one little boy so unbearably anxious that he stopped coming to school altogether.

Nathan leads us past a series of low-rise glass buildings that look like greenhouses but don't appear to contain anything. A small bird has somehow found its way inside one of the structures and is flying happily from beam to beam, oblivious to its confinement. Nathan talks, explaining our surroundings, but we don't bother listening. We've learned not to rely on what he says.

'Here we are, Laurie-Amelia,' he announces as we arrive at a set of large steel gates set into a high wire-mesh fence, the top of which curls sharply outward.

Benjamin-Annie's in here?

He enters a code into the keypad on the gate and scans his ID badge. He extends his hand. 'I need yours too.'

'Mine?'

'Your ID card.' He nods at our lanyard.

'Oh.' We take it off and pass it to him. We've never needed to use our card for access before. We'd forgotten that's what it's for.

He scans the card, and there's the sound of the gate unlocking. A soft click. It shuts smoothly and silently behind us. Through a screen of fir trees, we make out a cluster of pretty little houses, like something from a greetings card. We put our lanyard back on and follow Nathan down the shiny cobblestone path. We glance back at the fence, its sharp edges promising pain to anyone who dares to climb it.

We emerge onto a street lined with charming red-brick houses, each with a neatly manicured lawn and green picket fence. It's as though we've stepped onto the set of a suburban drama, where everyone wears cheerful smiles, and dark secrets lurk behind closed doors.

'Isn't it lovely?' Nathan says. 'Each house is home to two Support Workers and two Combines of a similar age. It helps with the children's recovery, you know, to feel part of a nuclear unit. There's a very special sense of community within The Enclave. Can you imagine a child trying to adjust to their merged self in an apartment like yours? It wouldn't be fair. They need the space, the gardens, the family dynamic.'

We pass a Support Worker tending to a window box. They hum softly as they carefully deadhead the flowers that have gone over, too absorbed in their work to notice us. 'Does Benjamin-Annie have a house?' we ask.

'They do indeed,' Nathan says. 'Though they don't share their house with another Combine. Just Angela. They're an anomaly, being the only adult Combine living here. And little Teddy is, of course, the only newborn.'

Ahead of us, a toddler no older than three, with a head of dark, curly hair, walks hand in hand with a Support Worker, their little fingers pointing excitedly at our balloon. 'Cloud,' they say proudly.

'That's right,' the Support Worker says. 'A cloud. Very good, Nathaniel-Rose. There aren't any clouds in the sky today, though.'

The child looks up, eyes scanning the clear sky as if double-checking the truth of what they've been told.

It's so strange to see a child Combine, and yet so common for children to be put forward for the Merge. So many families have no choice. They're like war horses, driven into battle with no say, no awareness of the life that lies ahead.

We expect to feel some fondness for the child, something beyond sympathy and guilt, but we don't. Our usual enthusiasm for children must be waning as we align.

Panic stirs. If our personality is fading, blending, are we too far along in our Merge to keep hold of our separate selves? To maintain two perspectives? We need both – we need to speak, to disagree, to see things differently.

We need each other.

'There's a large school here,' Nathan says, waving at Nathaniel-Rose's Support Worker as we pass. 'I can show it to you if you'd like. It has its own petting zoo. Are you thinking of getting back into teaching, Laurie-Amelia? Perhaps we could get you a position in the school here before you're signed off. It's never too soon to start getting back to your career.'

'I think I'd rather continue with the videography,' we say, surprising ourselves with the certainty of our statement. 'Twenty-five years of teaching is enough.'

Nathan nods. 'Quite understandable. Well, we can certainly get you filming again soon. Perhaps you could document little Teddy's Naming Ceremony.' We pass a front garden where two young Combines run and laugh. Nathan notices us watching and misreads the tension in our expression as admiration. 'It's lovely to witness, isn't it?' he says. 'Combine children are incredibly resilient compared to adults. They bounce back so quickly. They've fewer memories, you see, so less conflict.'

'What about the children who merge with adults? Do they live here, too?'

'Yes, they do. Although they share the mind of an elder, they remain very much a child in their life stage and are treated as such. It works the same both ways. You may well be sharing an apartment block with a Combine whose Transfer was a child. Though that's rarer, of course. Most people merge in… the other direction.'

Nathan stops outside the house we assume belongs to Benjamin-Annie. It's red brick, framed by a green picket fence. Identical to the others. 'Now,' he says, slipping his hands into his trouser pockets. 'There's something you need to know before we go inside.' He licks his lips, rocking back on his heels. 'Benjamin-Annie doesn't know about Lara-Jay.'

We blink at him, taken aback. 'What?'

'They gave birth just a couple of hours after Lara-Jay died. They haven't had it easy, Laurie-Amelia, as I'm sure they'll tell you. Becoming a parent has been a huge adjustment for them. So, Angela made the executive decision that they shouldn't be told. Not until they're ready.'

We tilt our head, our eyes lingering on the picket fence. We can't begin to imagine what they've been through. Perhaps it's sensible to spare them from more grief, to allow them to navigate these fragile first weeks without added strain. *But what happens when they find out? When they realise everyone knew and chose to keep them in the dark?*

Mum?

Nothing comes.

'Just be there for them,' Nathan says. 'Show them love, support and understanding. Keep conversations light and focus on Teddy. Trust that Angela has their best interests at heart. When the time is right, they'll know about everything that has been happening. Until then, we do our best to support them and protect their new family. Okay?'

We nod. 'Okay.'

Nathan knocks loudly on the door.

We fidget with the string of the balloon. This is it. Our reunion with Benjamin-Annie. The first time we'll meet their son. They'll open the door, Teddy cradled in their arms, his little face wide-eyed and innocent. Benjamin-Annie will smile, or maybe they'll hesitate, taking us in, getting used to our presence before deciding to let us inside.

But the door remains closed. No soft footsteps, no murmurs from inside, not even the faintest cry of a baby disturbed by the knock. We glance at Nathan, who's chewing his lip. 'They probably need a minute,' he says. 'Don't worry.'

I have a bad feeling. Do you? I don't think they're here. And Nathan will say they've popped out, that we can come back tomorrow. But then we'll come back tomorrow and—

The door opens, and there they are.

Benjamin-Annie.

We release a breath of relief and step forward to embrace them, holding them so tightly they let out a soft laugh. They're okay. They're here, and in this moment they seem happy. We eventually loosen our hold on them and pass them the balloon. 'Here,' we say. 'Congratulations. I can't believe it. You're a parent now. You did it, Benjamin-Annie. You've started your family.'

They take the balloon, their smile warm but distant, their eyes lifting to the cloud-shaped message floating above. 'So happy,' they say, their head tilting slightly, as if contemplating the statement. Their red curls are longer than they were last time we saw them, but just as wild. Something about them is different, though, something subtle. *It's their makeup, the lack of it.* We nod. That's what it is. The rosy blush that used to tint their cheeks is gone. Perhaps that's Ben's influence. Perhaps he isn't comfortable wearing makeup.

'Congratulations,' we say again, though our voice falters this time, thickened by the sudden undeniable awareness of Ben standing before us, seeing us through Annie's eyes. 'It's so good to see you, Benjamin-Annie. I've been so worried. How are you?'

Angela appears behind them. She hurries past Benjamin-Annie to embrace us, kissing us twice on both cheeks. 'Oh, Laurie-Amelia,' she says. 'It's so lovely to see you. You look so well.'

'You do,' Benjamin-Annie says. 'You look beautiful.'

We smile, but it isn't true. Our hair, once thick and shiny, is now brittle and thinning, and no matter how hard we try, we can't seem to put any weight on. Our clothes hang loosely on our too-thin frame. But it's a kind thing for them to say. And it's such a relief to hear them speak. To see them standing here, so healthy and strong.

'Come on in,' Angela says. 'Come and meet our delightful little man.'

We step inside and bend to take off our shoes. 'No, no,' Angela says. 'Don't worry about that. Keep them on.'

We look at Nathan, who nods reassuringly. Benjamin-Annie's house is immaculate. It feels wrong to be wearing our shoes, like spoiling fresh snow with our footprints. The place seems to gleam with cleanliness; every surface freshly polished, appearing untouched, as though no one lives here at all, especially not a newborn.

Our mind begins to race. Is this truly Benjamin-Annie's home, or just the place Nathan wants us to believe they've been all this time? We replay the wait at the door, the way the minutes dragged. Why did it take so long for Benjamin-Annie to answer?

A new, unsettling thought takes hold. We picture Angela ushering them in moments before we arrived, scrambling to pull them from their real home – a space cluttered with toys, baby bottles, nappies and piles of tiny clothes – and placing them here, in this sterile environment, just in time to put on a convincing show. The idea of The Enclave being nothing more than a set, and this house nothing more than a carefully curated prop, creeps back.

'Your house is beautiful,' we say.

Benjamin-Annie smiles, leading us to the nursery. The balloon trails behind them, bouncing from the ceiling. *So Happy!* 'Thank you,' they say.

'It's very tidy.'

They nod. 'Cleaning helps me.'

'Helps you?'

We pass rows of photos in matching silver frames, perfectly straight and evenly spaced along the walls. Images of Ben and Annie, of their pregnancy shoot, of their friends and family. There's a shot of them at their Commitment Ceremony, hand in hand in their purple robes. We stop in front of the image, staring at it, straining for a memory to surface, but nothing comes. We touch the frame. 'Do you remember that day, Benjamin-Annie? Do you remember Committing?'

They turn and see us touching their photograph. Their eyes widen, and they let go of the balloon. 'Don't touch,' they say, hurrying over and using their sleeve to wipe the frame where our fingers have been.

'Sorry,' we say. 'I shouldn't have touched it. I'm sorry, Benjamin-Annie.'

They don't respond. They're frantically wiping the frame.

The freed balloon floats up the stairwell and vanishes into the shadows above.

We look at Nathan. 'It's okay, Laurie-Amelia,' Angela says gently. 'Benjamin-Annie can be rather – particular. That's all. It's nothing personal. Come on through to the nursery. We'll let Benjamin-Annie get things sorted, and you can meet darling little Teddy. He's just delightful.'

We follow her, casting a backwards glance as Benjamin-Annie carefully removes the photo frame from the wall.

'Here we are,' Angela says.

We stare, frowning at the nursery. *Am I going mad, or... is this room identical to the nursery at their apartment?* 'The walls,' we say. 'They're pink and orange. It looks just like...'

Angela nods, smiling. 'I had their old nursery replicated. Everything's the same, right down to the rug.' She walks over to the crib. We follow slowly, taking in our surroundings. There's the wicker toybox, the low chest of drawers, the white-laced crib. The sight transports us back to the original nursery, to the time we were there, standing by the crib, convinced we were pregnant.

Feeling that level of confusion doesn't seem possible now. *How far we've come.*

A faint whimper rises from the crib. We hold back, closing our eyes, bracing ourselves for the sight of the child Ben and Annie so desperately wanted, the child they've risked everything to bring into this world. We've been longing for this moment since we first heard about him, but now that it's here it's almost too much to bear.

'Come on, Laurie-Amelia,' Angela says gently. 'Come and meet Teddy.'

We take a deep breath before opening our eyes. We approach the crib slowly, waiting until we're right up close before allowing ourselves to look. We gasp. Teddy is so tiny, wrapped in a green woollen blanket and wearing a cotton hat embroidered with the Combine mandala. His tiny hands are covered in green mittens, and his tiny chest rises and falls with each breath.

A miracle.

'He's pretty amazing, isn't he?'

We turn, our eyes watering. Benjamin-Annie is standing by the doorway, smiling. 'Hold him,' they say. 'Please. He's in need of some love.'

Angela tucks one hand gently under Teddy's back, the other under his head, and scoops him up. 'Teddy,' she says. 'Meet Laurie-Amelia.' She places him in our arms. His warmth sinks into us. We trace his cheek with a trembling finger, and our tears fall. It's been so long since we felt the delicate softness of newborn skin. We'd almost forgotten how impossibly small and fragile a baby can feel. He blinks sleepily up at us, his lips twitching. We kiss his tiny nose, overwhelmed by the love we feel for him.

Our love for babies is still here. We're still here.

'He's absolutely perfect, Benjamin-Annie,' we say. 'You've done so well.'

We rock Teddy to sleep as Benjamin-Annie fills us in on what's been happening with them. They sit cross-legged on the rug, their curls falling around their face as they absent-mindedly smooth out the rug's wrinkles and creases. 'I was finding everything okay in the beginning,' they say. 'I was excited. Being surrounded by all the children felt like the perfect preparation. But then I started to get all panicky. I was worrying about the challenges of doing this alone, of raising a baby with one body as opposed to two.' They clear their throat, smoothing down the rug's pile so that it all goes in the same direction. 'I'd thought about it before, of course I had. But it suddenly seemed overwhelming. I put it down to the hormones and told myself I'd feel calmer once the baby arrived. But when Teddy came, I had this episode…'

They look at Angela, who's leaning against the wall by the crib. She stands beside Nathan. Both have their arms folded. Nathan looks especially uncomfortable.

'Can I tell Laurie-Amelia what happened?'

'Of course you can, Benjamin-Annie,' Angela says. 'You can tell Laurie-Amelia whatever you please, so long as you feel up to it.'

Benjamin-Annie begins smoothing the rug again, their fingers creating small paths. It's a while before they look at us through the curtain of curls. 'I went mad, Laurie-Amelia. I lost my mind. I screamed at poor Angela whenever she came near Teddy. I kept accusing her of wanting to steal him. I believed it, too. I really believed she was going to take him from me. I only recently came to my senses. It's terrifying when you realise you've gone insane.'

'You were never insane, Benjamin-Annie,' Angela says. 'You were suffering from post-partum psychosis. That's nothing to be ashamed of.'

'Oh, Benjamin-Annie,' we say, our voice soft with regret. 'I'm so sorry I wasn't around to help you through that.'

They shake their head, their eyes on Teddy. A tiny yawn escapes his mouth, as if to assure them that nothing has troubled him. He's still perfectly content. 'I'm really pleased you didn't see me in that state. I'd probably have accused you of wanting Teddy for yourself, too.'

'Do you want him back?' we ask, suddenly aware of how long he's been in our arms.

They shake their head again, returning their attention to the rug. 'I don't hold him anymore.'

We look at Angela and Nathan, both wearing the same sad expression.

'I don't trust myself,' Benjamin-Annie whispers. 'Having two parents in one body isn't right, isn't natural, it's too much, too strong, too... I'm scared I love him too much and that, if I hold him, I'll squeeze him too tightly and suffocate him.' They shuffle backwards, retreating from the intensity of their own affection. 'It's better this way. It means he'll be safe.'

Oh, god. I can't stand it.

'He'll be safe with you, Benjamin-Annie. I'm sure of it.'

They smile weakly. 'That's kind of you to say, but if you'd seen me... Did you feel crazy after you gave birth? Did you ever worry you'd hurt Amelia?'

We pause, trying to sift through the jumble in our head. The worry in their eyes makes us want to give them something to hold on to. Our gaze wanders, searching the air as if the answer might be floating around, waiting to be caught. We feel the strain of the effort, like reaching into a fog. 'I felt delirious with love,' we say. 'I'd spend the nights watching her, guarding her as she slept. I was terrified, just as you are. I had this need to protect her from everything. Even when Mitchell, her father, would hold her, I couldn't properly relax. The only time I felt I could breathe easily was when she was in my arms.'

Teddy's properly awake now, babbling happily in our arms. We gently bounce him, admiring his bright eyes and toothless grin. 'He's got your eyes, Ben,' we say. 'I was hoping he would.'

Benjamin-Annie is polishing the perfectly clean windowsills. 'Tell me about the others,' they say, pausing to observe their work before deciding it's not up to standard and resuming their wiping.

We tense, and Teddy squeezes our fingers tightly, still gazing up at us. 'Noah-Lucas is doing really well,' we say. 'They're so healthy. They're loving life as a Combine. They go to school and everything, and they've got tons of energy. It's so wonderful to see.'

Benjamin-Annie smiles. 'I'll have to invite them over,' they say, finally putting the cloth down. 'Angela's only allowing me one visitor a day and, selfishly perhaps, I wanted to see you first. Maybe Noah-Lucas should come next time. How about Lara-Jay? Are they coping? I've been thinking about them a lot. It can't be easy for them. It's been difficult enough for me, and we were in love.'

Teddy kicks his little legs energetically, as though urging us on. 'They're not out of their apartment yet,' we say quickly, 'so can't say for sure. But from what I hear, they're doing well.' We force a laugh. 'Looks like you've got a little kickboxer here.'

'Tell me about it. He was in training long before he was born. It was the most surreal feeling, like he was trying to communicate with me, warn me about something.' They watch his busy legs. 'Teddy's being presented to the world next week. Did Nathan tell you?'

We shake our head.

'At your signing-off party,' Nathan explains. 'Little Teddy is the guest of honour.'

Benjamin-Annie's eyes are fixed on their son. 'I don't know how it will go. Angela says I'll have to hold him.'

'It won't be for long,' Angela reassures, 'just for the photographs. The world wants to celebrate your miracle, Benjamin-Annie. And they can't do that if they don't see you with your baby.'

Benjamin-Annie picks the cloth up and starts wiping again, a repetitive, almost frantic motion.

We travel to the party with Benjamin-Annie, Noah-Lucas and the Support Workers. Teddy sleeps peacefully in his car seat as Angela drives. We envy his innocence, his unawareness, his ability to drift off at a time like this. We stifle a yawn, staring out of the window at the first glimmers of daylight. We were woken well before sunrise, ushered into the van while it was still dark, our senses dulled by disrupted sleep.

Our sleep has been steadily deteriorating. Nathan tells us it's normal to have restless nights before being signed off, attributing it to the excitement. We are excited to get back to Albie, to Mary, to resume our real life – but we're also terrified. At night, we lie awake, contemplating the very real possibility that we have ventured too far down this path, that our minds are too intertwined to ever get our head-talk back to normal.

We should have been prepared for the quiet; we knew this lessening of head-talk would happen eventually. Nathan keeps reminding us that it's a sign of harmony, of alignment. But it's been weeks without any real conversation.

We're not ready to abandon each other. Not ready to say goodbye. Not yet.

Last night's sleep was the worst so far. Each time we drifted off, we were jolted awake, certain there was someone in the room, calling our name. Our old name. Amelia. The sound stirred something deep within us. We felt that pull, that silent tug-of-war that happens so frequently now. It was comforting to hear our old name, but the absence of the other name carried a quiet, lingering guilt.

Benjamin-Annie yawns loudly beside us, their head resting on our shoulder, their eyes closed. They've been murmuring their lines for most of the journey, quietly rehearsing their speech. We rest our head against theirs, unable to shake the image of them buckling under the weight of so many eyes.

'Why is Benjamin-Annie speaking at our signing-off party?' we asked Nathan when we first heard they'd be giving a talk. 'They've scarcely spent any time beyond The Enclave. Don't you think it'll overwhelm them being put in front of a crowd?'

Nathan rubbed his face in that familiar way, the one that signals a difficult response is coming. 'Actually, Laurie-Amelia, this party isn't just for you. Noah-Lucas and Benjamin-Annie are being signed off, too. Remember,' he added quickly, before we could protest, 'they will still be monitored and kept safe. Combine wants to celebrate the three of you. You're cured of Alzheimer's, Noah-Lucas is free of cancer, and Benjamin-Annie is a healthy parent to their healthy son. You've all succeeded. All of your trials have been successful. It wouldn't be fair to leave Benjamin-Annie behind, would it?'

We swallowed our objections, knowing they'd fall on deaf ears. Still, a quiet unease settled over us: If we aren't sure we're ready to leave The Village, then Benjamin-Annie most certainly isn't. *Why would they rush them like this?*

We waited, but no response came. No head-talk was needed. We already knew the answer: Combine needs to prove that the other experiments worked, that, although two lives were lost, others were saved and, in Benjamin-Annie's case, *created*.

Benjamin-Annie isn't just giving a speech today. They have the added pressure of introducing Teddy to the world, sitting on a panel to discuss the future of sustainable reproduction and Combine families.

'Are you sure you don't want to take part in any extra talks, Laurie-Amelia?' Nathan asked. 'Is there a panel you'd like to join? I don't want you missing out.'

We shook our head. 'I'm happy with the speech. Anything more might be too much. What if I blank and forget something, make everyone look bad?'

Nathan nodded, agreeing that we were wise to err on the side of caution. He passed us a copy of the speech he'd written and printed, and we scanned it. 'It's important that your words accurately reflect the success of your Merge,' he said. 'This is your opportunity to finish what you've started, to offer hope to millions living with Alzheimer's.'

We don't believe in what we'll be saying.

We don't believe we've been cured.

This is just the final step. The party comes before our release from The Village. If we do this, we can leave. And when we're out, we can finally speak the truth.

We'll tell Albie about the gaps in our memory that have never filled, no matter how often Nathan reassured us that they would. About Lara-Jay and how unfair it was to push them through the Merge when they were never ready. About all the times we were held inside, forced to comply, bullied into silence under the threat of losing our privileges.

We'll tell him how Lara and Jay's deaths are the fault of Combine, and Combine alone.

Noah-Lucas seems to be the only one with any energy. They've been happily chatting with the Support Workers about how great it feels to be out of The Village, marvelling at cars filled with regular people who have no idea we're Combines. 'I can't believe this is finally happening,' they say. 'We actually get to see what Combine life is like on the outside.'

We don't bother pointing out that today won't provide a realistic glimpse of life outside The Village, that we'll be surrounded by Combine supporters, everyone there to celebrate us, with no anti-Mergers in sight. Noah-Lucas wouldn't listen even if we did. They'd just shake their head knowingly and regurgitate the lines we've been fed. 'Combine supporters outnumber anti-Mergers, so it *is* accurate in its own way.'

We've been taking turns with Noah-Lucas to visit Benjamin-Annie. They can still only manage one visitor a day, so we divide our time fairly. We find ourselves jealous on Noah-Lucas's days, imagining the fun they're having, the jokes they're sharing. And yet, on our days, we can't shake the worry that our visits are more of a burden than a comfort. We aren't as good at lifting Benjamin-Annie's spirits.

'If they struggle with two visitors a day,' we asked Nathan, 'how will they manage at a party? How will they cope once they're outside The Village?'

Nathan frowned. 'I thought you trusted our judgement, Laurie-Amelia.'

'I just don't understand how they can be expected to—'

'Did I not make it clear that maintaining a consistently positive outlook is a requirement for attending the party? If you're still doubting Combine, then perhaps you're not ready to go home.'

We shook our head. 'You did. I'm sorry. I was just curious.'

Benjamin-Annie lifts their head from our shoulder and leans forward to check on Teddy. Angela notices in her rear-view mirror and smiles. 'How are you feeling?' she asks.

'I'm okay.'

'Not too nervous?'

'No,' they say. 'Excited, actually.'

We glance at them. We weren't expecting excitement. Neither, it seems, was Nathan, who raises his eyebrows with a slight chuckle. 'Good for you, Benjamin-Annie.'

'Just remember,' Angela says, her eyes still on the rear-view mirror, 'if you're in the middle of your speech and you get nervous or start to panic, you can take a break. You can always go to a separate room for some alone time. You don't need to be in the thick of it. No one expects you to be.'

Benjamin-Annie nods, settling back in their seat.

'And you, Laurie-Amelia?' Angela asks. 'Are you excited?'

We pause to consider this. There's a definite flutter in our stomach, but it feels more like anxiety than excitement. A tight, uneasy kind of anticipation. 'Yes,' we say, forcing a small nod. 'I am.'

'I feel bad for Lara-Jay,' Benjamin-Annie says. 'I know how it feels knowing that everyone is together without you. It's not nice. They'll be out of their apartment soon, right, Angela? Then they can join in the fun.'

'Yes. They'll be out soon. Don't worry about them, Benjamin-Annie. They don't know you're celebrating today.'

We swallow hard, focusing our attention out of the window, the passing scenery blurring

'Angela's right,' Noah-Lucas says. 'Today is a celebration, not a time to be worrying. Let's enjoy it, shall we?'

By the time we arrive at Alexandra Palace, it's full daylight. The grand building crowns the hill, its arched windows glinting in the morning sun. Green and purple banners cascade from the palace's facade, emblazoned with bold letters: **CONGRATULATIONS, COMBINES!**

Angela avoids the main entrance, where photographers cluster, their camera flashes bursting bright and blinding even against the sunlight.

She drives down a designated road leading to a discreet side entrance, bypassing the press gathered beneath the rose window.

A well-dressed team of security guards greets us and escorts us through the side entrance into a secluded hallway. The noise of the crowd outside fades to a distant hum. We're led into a private room with high ceilings and a mirror spanning across one wall. A large table sits in the centre, covered in makeup palettes, styling tools and rows of neatly arranged hair products.

A young woman, silent and avoiding eye contact, styles our hair and applies our makeup with quick, practised movements. Beside us, Teddy sits snug in his carrier, his tiny hand curled tightly around our little finger. He's dressed for the occasion in a Combine-green babygrow and his little mandala hat.

Benjamin-Annie sits in the chair next to ours, murmuring their lines while their hair is styled. They're too focused to talk, their lips moving faintly as they rehearse.

'Don't stress if you can't remember everything we've practised,' Angela says gently. 'The goal is to show what's possible, to give hope to anyone who wants to start a family. To prove that it's achievable without increasing the population.'

Benjamin-Annie nods. 'I know,' they say quietly. 'I just want to get it right.'

There's a knock on the door.

A man strides in. His head dips in a practised bow, his thick silver hair catching the light as he thanks us for our sacrifice. We recognise him instantly. Timothy Brightwell, Combine's lead investor. His face is everywhere – on ads, in magazines, across countless TV interviews.

He's made it clear, time and time again, that without him, Combine wouldn't exist, let alone thrive. The UK wouldn't be leading this mission to save the world. His message is unambiguous: without his money and vision, the world would be doomed.

Anger courses through us at the sight of him. His name flashes in our mind, plastered across placards, chanted in unison by furious crowds: *'FUCK COMBINE. FUCK BRIGHTWELL. FUCK COMBINE. FUCK BRIGHTWELL.'*

We remember the roar of approval when his makeshift effigy went up in flames. His face, smug and self-satisfied, was the embodiment of everything we despised. Slogans painted in bold, angry strokes screamed out his greed and manipulation.

The memory burns hot, rushing back in vivid flashes.

We clench our fists, nails digging into our palms to keep from lashing out.

We follow Noah-Lucas and Benjamin-Annie's lead, stepping into line to greet him. Brightwell moves along the row, extending his hand to each of us with a practised smile that doesn't reach his eyes. His teeth gleam unnaturally white, too bright for comfort. 'It's a real honour to meet you all,' he says.

We can hardly look at him, this man who has profited from our stories, our struggles, our very lives. This man who treats merging like a commodity, cashing in even in the wake of Lara-Jay's death.

Our stomach twists as Noah-Lucas beams and tells Mr Brightwell what an honour it is to meet him, to be in his presence. Brightwell smiles, returning the sentiment. 'Everyone is so extraordinarily excited to celebrate you three today.'

Teddy babbles softly in his carrier. Brightwell shakes his head, laughing lightly. 'Sorry. How incredibly rude of me. The *four* of you.' He turns to Benjamin-Annie. 'May I?'

They nod, and Brightwell approaches Teddy. He crouches in front of the carrier, shaking his head in exaggerated awe. 'Absolutely remarkable. The world's first Combine baby. You must be extraordinarily proud, Benjamin-Annie.'

Benjamin-Annie nods again, remaining silent, seemingly too stunned to speak.

Brightwell straightens and turns back to us. 'You *four* are our guests of honour. This party is for you. There's no obligation to do anything more than let us celebrate you, let us properly express our gratitude for everything you've done.'

He begins outlining the party's itinerary – live entertainment, a schedule of talks and demonstrations. 'Thirty-minute slots,' he says, 'have been allocated to each of you. There's no pressure to fill them, but the opportunity is there if you want it. I'm conscious that, for all of you, this is your first time out of The Village. No one expects perfection.' He flashes his insufferable smile. 'Any questions?'

Benjamin-Annie clears their throat. 'Is it absolutely necessary that Teddy is on stage with me?' they ask. 'During the panel session, I mean. I'm fine with having photographs taken, but I don't want to overwhelm him with all the noise and lights.'

'Everyone is dying to see Teddy,' Brightwell says. 'If you are on the panel, then it's essential he's there with you. He needn't stay the whole time. A brief appearance will suffice. After that, you, or your Support Worker, can bring him back here and stay with him until the party is over. Would that be acceptable?'

Benjamin-Annie nods, their shoulders relaxing slightly. 'Thank you.'

'Not at all.' Brightwell smiles. 'After your speeches, there will be a formal ceremony where you will be officially recognised and honoured for your achievements.'

This is the first we've heard of any ceremony. We frown at Nathan, who assured us he'd told us exactly what was going to be happening today.

He winks back at us, as if it's a harmless surprise.

The foyer buzzes with excitement. Food stalls offering a variety of cuisines line the space, and tables overflow with desserts that look almost too beautiful to eat. Throughout the venue, interactive exhibits showcase our achievements, our merging journeys displayed for all to see.

We stand with Nathan, observing Noah-Lucas as they hold court by their exhibit. They stand before a screen replaying

CCTV footage of their first bike ride, captivating the crowd with their anecdotes, just as they did in their interview. They pose for photos, draping their arms round strangers as though they're old friends, leaning in close as guests reach out to touch the mandala on their neck.

'Do you want to see your exhibit, Laurie-Amelia?' Nathan asks. 'There's some lovely footage of you. And your artwork is proudly displayed, of course.'

We shake our head. Our attention has been caught by a group of guests wearing virtual reality headsets. 'What're they doing?'

'Experiencing a day in the life of a Combine,' Nathan says. 'They'll be wandering around The Village, I expect.'

The upbeat rhythm of a live band fills the foyer as suited waiters weave through the crowd, expertly balancing trays of champagne flutes. Nearby, a photo booth with quirky props and backdrops attracts a steady stream of guests. We watch a woman rummage through the props before triumphantly selecting a pair of oversized sunglasses and a sign that reads *I MERGED*.

In the centre of the foyer, a large screen displays a ticking countdown. 'What's that for?' we ask, nodding towards it.

'It's counting down to the highlight of the evening,' Nathan says.

'The ceremony?'

He smiles and shakes his head, then gestures towards the far wall where a massive banner proclaims **COMBINE GOES GLOBAL**

'In precisely five hours and twenty-three minutes, everyone around the world will have access to the Merge, Laurie-Amelia. It's being rolled out worldwide. Isn't it fantastic?'

'What?'

He grins. 'You've caused waves, Laurie-Amelia. Now that you've proven merging can cure illnesses, everyone wants a piece. Your influence is going to be felt across the globe.'

We stare at the banner as faint applause rises in the distance.

It feels more like an indictment than a celebration.

All those people who will sign up, believing they can rid themselves of Alzheimer's. All because we were so desperate to leave The Village, and not brave enough to speak up.

We open our mouth to protest, to plead the roll-out doesn't go ahead, but the words falter. A sudden doubt grips us as we realise: We can't remember the last thing we forgot.

Is Combine right? Have we remembered everything? Could we actually be cured?

We close our eyes, imploring a response, straining for the faintest murmur of head-talk.

But there's nothing. Only silence.

An announcement crackles overhead, informing us that the Sustainable Parenthood Panel will commence in ten minutes. Nathan escorts us to the grand hall, where the stage is set for our presentation. The speaker currently onstage commands the room effortlessly, their voice steady, the audience still, captivated.

A prickling heat rises on our skin.

We could hold their attention too. We could use our time up there to reveal the truth, to finally voice what's been gnawing at us – to tell the world that we don't feel cured, that pieces of our memory are still missing.

But is that even true anymore? Every detail of this past week is sharp, clear. No haze, no confusion.

We think back further, to the days surrounding our Merge, and... nothing.

That emptiness, it's evidence, isn't it?

We catch the tail end of the live demonstration. The speaker explains how the watches are now updated to track mood and satisfaction levels in Combines, a measure designed to prevent future tragedies. It's something, at least. A small, belated acknowledgement of Lara-Jay. Some action taken in their name.

As the demonstration concludes, more people flood into the hall. Reporters from all over the world crowd in, their voices mingling in a cacophony of languages. Though we can't decipher much of what's being said, their excitement is unmistakable. The air hums with energy, a sense of eager anticipation filling the room.

The lights dim. Uniformed security guards, stationed strategically around the hall, monitor the crowd for any signs of trouble. The music softens, then disappears altogether as the panel files in.

They take their place at a long table, each seat marked by a bold name plaque. *Dr Sebastian Harrington: Lead Combine Scientist*; *Timothy Brightwell: Investor and co-owner, Combine Ltd*; *Benjamin-Annie Miller: Combine and Parent of Teddy Miller*; *Dr Edith Sinclaire: Genetics Expert*; *Professor Isabella Reynolds: Neurology Specialist*; *Kelly Parkins: Ethical Advisor*; *Winston-Adelaide Whittaker: Our Combine.*

We gasp, turning to Nathan. 'You didn't tell me that Our Combine would be here. I thought they weren't doing any more interviews.'

His mouth curves into a faint smile. 'An occasion as special as this warrants their presence, don't you think?'

The cameras must already be rolling. At the podium, Brightwell addresses the audience, his practised, artificial smile firmly in place. 'Esteemed guests, viewers from around the globe, it is my great privilege to stand before you today and present Combine's greatest achievement to date.'

He gestures towards Benjamin-Annie, who attempts a smile, but their jaw is tight, their expression stiff, more a strained grimace than a smile.

'Come on, Benjamin-Annie,' Nathan mutters. 'Relax.'

'During the long journey of pregnancy, Benjamin-Annie made the extraordinary choice to merge. It was a selfless, courageous act that we hoped, but could not be certain, would pay off. Today, we celebrate the success of their decision to undergo a Merge while pregnant. Today, I introduce to you Teddy Benjamin Miller. The world's first baby born from a Combine.'

Angela steps onto the stage, cradling Teddy carefully in her arms.

For a moment, the crowd is silent, stunned. Then cheers erupt, excited applause rippling through the hall. We hold our breath as Benjamin-Annie stands and takes their son from Angela.

They manage it.

They hold him gently to their chest and smile.

Cameras are raised. Rapid bursts of light fill the room. We watch as Benjamin-Annie tries to maintain their composure, blinking rapidly in the brightness. We squint, blinded on their behalf, as Brightwell resumes his speech. 'The birth of this precious child brings with it a cascade of questions, wonder and, undoubtedly, a medley of emotions. Today, we will delve into the ethical considerations, the rigorous safeguards implemented, and the collaborative efforts that brought forth this glorious moment in history.'

The flashes continue, relentless and greedy. 'Surely they have enough now,' we say to Nathan. 'How many photos do they need?'

'We extend our gratitude to the global community for their curiosity, support and open-mindedness. Together, we stand at the threshold of a bold new era.'

The flashing finally ceases. Benjamin-Annie sinks back into their seat, relief washing over their face.

The grand hall quiets, the air still buzzing with the echoes of applause. We watch Benjamin-Annie, still cradling Teddy, their hands gentle but unsteady. Someone was supposed to take him backstage, to carry him away from the lights and eyes of the crowd. Why is he still there?

Nathan leans in close, his breath warm against our ear. 'This is your moment too, Laurie-Amelia. Remember that.'

We nod. Swallow. The world is watching, and we don't have long to decide what to say.

We could follow Nathan's script, play the part and get home to Albie. Once we're safely out of here, we could share the truth. Or we could speak up now, warn Alzheimer's patients against merging, and risk the walls closing in on us all over again.

If only we were clearer on what we actually remember.

Somehow, Teddy remains quiet through all of this, no tears, no fuss. It's as though he instinctively understands that his silence is the only thing keeping Benjamin-Annie from spiralling. We lean forward, trying to get a better view.

Is Teddy asleep? He can't have slept through all of that, surely.

Nothing.

The discussion begins, the panellists delving into the ethical implications and the scientific triumphs of the Merge. We try to focus, to absorb the information, in case something important slips past us. But it's difficult to stay present.

'...and explore the future,' Dr Harrington is saying, 'that we can now expect to enjoy, a world in which new life is no longer frowned upon, no longer judged, or viewed as a sinful act, a world in which the joy of new life aligns seamlessly with our responsibility to preserve and protect our planet.'

Benjamin-Annie gazes down at their son as Dr Harrington drones on, their focus entirely on Teddy. As if the rest of the world has faded away. When the presentation finally ends, and the floor is opened for questions, they blink at the crowd, momentarily startled, as though they'd forgotten where they were.

Every reporter's hand shoots up. Microphones are passed to a select few. The process is meticulous. There's no push-back on any of the answers the reporters receive. No squabbling, no impatience.

'Owen Tredgold from *America Today*,' a young reporter in the front row says when the microphone is handed to him. 'Can you elaborate on the potential long-term effects on Teddy's neurological development, being the child of a Combine? Are there any concerns regarding potential consequences?'

Professor Reynolds takes the question. 'We have conducted extensive research on the possible long-term effects of the merging process on neurological development. Our findings, based on initial observations, suggest that Teddy's neural connectivity aligns within the typical ranges. Of course, rigorous and continuous monitoring, along with a comprehensive programme of further study, will be conducted to ensure solutions are rapidly found for any potential issues. Let us not forget that we are very much working at the frontiers of science here.'

Throughout, Benjamin-Annie holds Teddy close, their arms wrapped protectively around him.

The microphone is passed to Caroline Halbrook from the BBC. 'My question is for Our Combine, Winston-Adelaide.' She bows her head, holding the gesture longer than she would for any other Combine. 'Thank you for your sacrifice. As the inaugural Combine, I was wondering what your personal view is on merging and sustainable parenthood?'

Our Combine pauses, their expression unreadable as they gather their thoughts. We lean in slightly, torn between conflicting emotions. We despise them for what they've started, for the path they paved that we felt compelled to follow. And yet, having endured the process ourselves, we can't help but feel a grudging respect. Never did we imagine we'd see them in person, much less witness them speak.

They lower their head slowly towards the microphone. Their movements, like their words, are deliberate, unhurried. It's how they've been since their Merge, a trait we once assumed all Combines would share. But Our Combine is unique. It adds to their allure, their strange, magnetic power; a reminder etched into every pause and measured word: They were the first.

'I believe what Combine has achieved in merging a pregnant Host with a Transfer is, quite simply, revolutionary. The merge of a pregnant woman not only addresses population concerns but allows for the guilt-free growth of families from hereon in. As such, it has my full endorsement.'

We scan the crowd. The audience is enthralled, hanging on every word from Our Combine. But the reporters exude a different energy, a calmness, as though they've seen this all before. They absorb everything with measured patience, pens poised over notepads, seemingly unruffled by the electric anticipation around them. It's almost as if they know the answers before they're spoken.

A microphone is passed to a reporter near the back of the room. 'Adrian Cornell from *The Times*. Benjamin-Annie...' He bows his head and thanks them for their sacrifice. 'Do you believe the merging process has influenced the bond between you and your child compared to the usual parenting experience?'

Benjamin-Annie shifts slightly, holding Teddy closer.

The room stills, waiting.

We're about to return our attention to the stage when we notice him, standing near the edge of the crowd. A young man wearing a black cap. We can't see his eyes, but it feels as if he's staring directly at us. Something about him – his posture, the tilt of his head – is familiar. We narrow our eyes, leaning forward again, but the shadow of the cap obscures his face.

'I've no prior experience of being a parent, so it's difficult to say. Impossible really…'

We shut our eyes tightly, and reopen them to a burst of coloured dots. We're still being watched.

But it isn't just him.

There's a woman, too. She isn't hidden beneath a cap, and her features are so familiar they steal our breath. *Eliza. It's her, isn't it? She's right there, staring at us.* Eliza leans in, whispering something in the man's ear. He nods, his head still angled towards us.

Benjamin-Annie's voice rises. 'Throughout the Preparation Period, we were told that merging was the coming together of two individuals to create something new. But…'

The young man raises a finger to his lips as Eliza's hand gently settles on his shoulder.

Albie.

Albie!

'Everything we were told was false.' Benjamin-Annie's voice rises over the murmurs in the hall. 'I was merging with my fiancé, Ben. We were supposed to live the rest of our lives together in my body. But it wasn't true… Nothing about me has changed. I don't have Ben's tastes, Ben's humour, Ben's knowledge. I can't feel him. I can't feel his love for our son. I can't hear him.' They take a steadying breath, but their voice wavers. 'The truth is that Ben, my fiancé, is no longer with us. I believe that he never merged with me. I believe that he has been taken by Combine, and now there's just me and Teddy.'

What?

Benjamin-Annie is shaking, the microphone trembling in their hand. The hall erupts in chaos. Frenzied voices rise, overlapping as questions come from every direction.

'Are you saying that you're not Ben, that you're only Annie?'

'Did you voice your concerns to anyone?'

'Are there others like you who believe their Partner has been taken?'

'What evidence do you have to support your claims?'

'Is this why Lara-Jay committed suicide?'

Benjamin-Annie's eyes widen in confusion, their head shaking. 'What? Did you say Lara-Jay killed—'

Security guards storm the stage, surrounding Benjamin-Annie and pulling Teddy from their arms. 'Don't let them take Teddy,' Benjamin-Annie screams, their voice cracking under the strain. 'Don't let them take him!'

As the guards drag Benjamin-Annie away, their cries reverberate, rising above the roar of the crowd. Their voice, hoarse and frantic, echoes through the hall.

'They took him. They took Ben. And now they're taking Teddy. Don't you see?'

We don't dream. We don't hear any intruders in the night. Our eyes open to the room gradually brightening. *Good morning, Combines. Remember, each sunrise is a blessing. Each day another opportunity to come closer to total alignment.*

A headache throbs.

We have no memory of our journey home. The last thing we recall is Albie running towards us, his mouth moving, forming words we couldn't hear. Couldn't make out.

And then we were bundled into the van.

We sit up slowly, the pounding in our head intensifying. There's a lump on our forehead. Unsteady, we push ourselves up to see the mirror. We lean in, examining the swelling, our fingertips brushing it cautiously. Pain flares. We flinch.

What happened?

We wait, listening. But there's nothing. No response. Just an empty silence.

Our eyes sting as tears fill them, spilling over. A release of the intense loneliness that's been building, quietly suffocating us for days.

We try again. *We saw Eliza. Do you remember? She was in the crowd. She was with Albie. What were they doing together?*

Nothing.

The announcement continues. *The Village is in lockdown.* No explanation is given, but we don't need one. Benjamin-Annie's statement has us sealed inside again. No sign-off, no homecoming. The ethereal voice remains calm as if everything is perfectly normal. *Remember, you are the future. You are the answer. You are the cure.*

How do we want to play this? We close our eyes, begging the head-talk to return, pleading for some response. Any response. *Do we act as though everything's fine? Or do we stand up to them and risk being locked inside again?*

'Good morning, Laurie-Amelia.'

We open our eyes. Nathan is standing beside our bed, watching us. He didn't knock.

'What's got you all upset?'

'I'm fine,' we say quickly. 'My head's a little sore, that's all.'

'Ah, yes. I'm afraid that's my fault.' He passes us a tissue, and we use it to wipe our nose. 'I panicked when the reporters were pursuing us. You tripped and fell. I'm dreadfully sorry.'

'It's fine,' we say. 'It's not too bad.'

His words trigger a memory – a blur of falling, the world spinning in slow motion, the ground rushing up. Then a sharp prick in our arm. And everything faded to black.

Nathan stays with us for breakfast. He doesn't eat, just sits across from us, watching.

We try to partake in head-talk, pushing as hard as we can for a response. But there's nothing. No murmur, no faint voice. *Did we dream it? Or was Albie actually there? He can't have been, can he? How would he have got in?*

We think of Benjamin-Annie, of their words: *The truth is that Ben, my fiancé, is no longer with us. I believe that he never merged with me. I believe that he has been taken by Combine, and now there's just me and Teddy.*

We remember every word. Word for word.

No confusion. No blanks.

If Combine has taken Ben, then where is he? What does it mean to be 'taken'?

Nothing.

With each failed attempt to communicate, the silence becomes more suffocating. Is this what happened to Ben and Annie? If so, are we next? Is Combine already making their move, slowly pulling Mum away, just like they did with Ben?

But Mum is here. We're both still here.

No one's been taken.

'You must have a lot of questions,' Nathan prompts. 'You're being awfully quiet.' His eyes remain fixed on us, his thumb absentmindedly rubbing the edge of the table. 'I'm so sorry you had to see Benjamin-Annie during a manic episode. This is why we kept them away for so long. We were trying to shield you from that experience.'

He has us. We need to know. 'What's going to happen to them?'

Nathan sighs loudly, the sound so familiar it triggers something raw inside us. We grip the edge of the chair, imagining it's him beneath our nails, his flesh giving way under the pressure. We dig our fingers in tight, picturing the pain he'd feel if it were really him.

'I was so hoping it wouldn't come to this,' he says, his voice so pathetic, so false. We clench our fists tighter, imagining the whiteness of our knuckles, the strain of restraint. 'I really hoped I'd never have to divulge the details about Teddy's birth and Benjamin-Annie's experience immediately afterwards, but it's important you understand. Otherwise, yesterday's episode will seem more harrowing than it needs to.'

He rubs his temples, thinking up a story, a tidy excuse that will explain all of this, brush it under the carpet, make it go away. 'As you know, Benjamin-Annie had a rough time after giving birth. You heard them call themselves mad. The thing is, Laurie-Amelia, they aren't mad. I urge you to remember that. No matter what they may seem, they aren't insane. They're just suffering from post-partum psychosis.'

We bite the inside of our cheek and taste blood.

'When I first visited Benjamin-Annie after they'd given birth to Teddy, they tried to attack me. They truly believed I'd taken Ben and intended to steal Teddy. It was terribly sad.' He shakes his head slowly. 'What's important to remember is that

Benjamin-Annie recovered once before, and they will recover again. Their distress and confusion is simply the result of a traumatic birth. Imagine it, Laurie-Amelia. Imagine giving birth as a Combine. It must have been dreadful experiencing all that pain, going through childbirth in a body that isn't entirely your own.'

We struggle to keep our voice steady, forcing down the rising anger. 'If their birth was so terrible, then why is it being celebrated as a success? And why was Benjamin-Annie paraded in front of all those people, all those cameras? If they were unwell, you should never have allowed it.'

'It wasn't my doing.'

'I didn't hear you voicing any concern. Did you tell them not to do it?'

His expression confirms what we already know. He didn't.

And now we're stuck here, too.

Eliza comes to our apartment that morning. When we open the door, her eyes dart past us, checking for Nathan. Before we can say a word, she pulls us into a tight embrace, her breath warm against our ear as she whispers. 'Please, don't say a word to Nathan. I'll explain everything.'

In the lounge, we sit together. Nathan, Eliza, and us.

Eliza's voice is calm as she tells us she witnessed what happened with Benjamin-Annie, as if we didn't already know she'd been there. 'You know there's no truth to it, don't you?' she says. 'No one wants to steal Teddy from his parent.'

'Laurie-Amelia understands,' Nathan assures her. 'They know what Benjamin-Annie's been through. I've told them everything.'

Eliza smiles, though it doesn't quite reach her eyes. 'Good. I just wanted to make sure.' She touches our arm gently. 'Can I make anyone a cup of tea?'

We take this as our cue, forcing a smile. 'I'd love one, thank you, Eliza. I'll help you.'

But Nathan follows us into the kitchen and leans against the counter with his arms folded as we get the mugs from the cupboard. Eliza fills the kettle. 'Oh, Nathan,' she says, 'Mike wanted you to give him a call. Something about house-arrest regulations.'

Nathan frowns, checking his watch. 'He hasn't contacted me.'

'He caught me on my way here. I told him I was coming over.'

Nathan hesitates, then pulls his phone from his pocket. Eliza puts the kettle on. We listen to the low rumble of water as it starts to heat.

Nathan dials. We glance at Eliza. If this is a bluff, she's about to be found out. But she looks calm, relaxed, her face serene as she waits for the kettle to boil.

'Mike?' Nathan says. 'Eliza said you wanted to speak to me? Something about house-arrest regulations?' He looks at us briefly, frowns. 'Yes, they are.' He nods, grunts, then holds up a finger, mouthing, *One moment.*

We hold our breath as he steps out of the room.

The moment the door closes, we rush to Eliza. 'You were with Albie,' we whisper. 'I saw you with him. You were whispering—'

'I can't explain now. There's no time,' she says quickly. 'But he wants you to know he hasn't given up, and that he won't give up. He told me to tell you to keep going, and that he's in touch with Lara-Jay's family. They're doing okay. I promised I'd get you through, and out of here. He'll be waiting.'

We glance at the door. Nathan's already wrapping up his call. 'Take me to Benjamin-Annie, Eliza. Let me check on them.'

'I'm working on getting you outside, Laurie-Amelia. That's what the phone—'

Nathan steps back into the kitchen. We move apart, the kettle whistling softly. Eliza pours the boiling water into the mugs, her hands remarkably steady, unlike ours. Our whole body is trembling.

'What was it about?' she asks. 'Is everything okay?'

Nathan nods, though his brow is furrowed. He guides Eliza aside, lowering his voice, trying and failing to keep us from hearing. 'He was updating me on the lockdown. It's been scrapped. He says keeping Laurie-Amelia inside could be detrimental to their mental well-being, that it's important they get fresh air, that their morale remains boosted for the remainder of their time here.'

'I see where he's coming from,' Eliza says, her voice equally low. 'We only need to look at Lara-Jay to understand what a depressive episode can do to a Combine. Keeping Laurie-Amelia happy is the right call, isn't it?'

'But it's so soon,' Nathan mutters. 'They've only just experienced—'

'I need a purpose,' we blurt out, louder than intended, the words spilling out in a rush. It's just like when we were a child, always giving ourselves away too easily.

Nathan's eyes widen.

'Sorry,' we say quickly, forcing a calmer tone. 'It's just, after seeing Benjamin-Annie yesterday, and knowing everything they've been through... I don't want to end up like them.'

Nathan's expression softens. 'You won't, Laurie-Amelia. I promise. That's not something you need to worry about.'

'But I am worried,' we press. 'I think I need something to focus on, something to occupy my mind. I see Noah-Lucas doing so well and I can't help but think it's because they have school to keep them busy.'

Eliza is watching us closely.

'You can't go to school, Laurie-Amelia,' Nathan says.

'Not to be a student, no. But I could teach. It's like you're always saying. I need to keep my options open. I'm not sure I'm up for taking on a class of my own, but maybe I could help out as a teaching assistant. I think that could be really good for me.'

There's silence. Nathan leans on the counter, his fingers tapping lightly as he considers our proposal. 'I suppose you could go in with Noah-Lucas,' he says eventually. 'You could assist in their class.'

Eliza removes the tea bags from the mugs and drops them in the bin. She moves casually, unhurried, but her eyes meet ours for a moment. A silent confirmation. She's with us. She understands.

'Isn't it primary school that you teach?' she asks, her voice conversational. 'I have a friend who works at the primary school here. I can get in touch, see if they need a hand in The Enclave.'

We nod eagerly. 'Yes please. Spending time with the little ones will keep me sane. I'm sure of it.'

'I think it's a brilliant idea,' Eliza says, turning to Nathan. 'We don't want Laurie-Amelia stuck inside, overthinking everything. It's like you always say, a busy mind is a healthy mind.'

'Yes,' Nathan says slowly. 'I suppose it is. Good for you, Laurie-Amelia.'

We turn away, hiding our smile.

Two days later, Nathan has a meeting and leaves us in Eliza's care. 'She's kindly arranged to take you to The Enclave to meet her friend who teaches at the school. You'll be given a tour and, if all goes well, we can get you signed up to work as an assistant.'

The waiting has been tortuous. We've tried to occupy ourselves, spending hours on thousand-piece puzzles and art therapy, but our thoughts remain trapped in an unrelenting loop, imagining the consequences Benjamin-Annie might face for their outburst, worrying about Teddy's well-being, and replaying the memory of Eliza and Albie, wondering why they were together, what they're planning, and why we're still being kept in the dark.

As we walk, Eliza talks, her voice low. She quietly instructs us on how to slip out of the school and find Benjamin-Annie's house. She'll stay behind in the school office, keeping her friend occupied. 'When you've been there, when you've seen them, you'll have a lot of questions. I'll answer them all. I'll tell you everything I know. But you need to see them first – for your own state of mind.' She touches our hand lightly. 'Stay hidden, Laurie-Amelia, and be quick.'

We nod, our stomach churning.

At the school, Eliza signs us in. The rather severe-looking middle-aged woman at the office informs us that her friend isn't working today. 'Teacher Abioye is in Monday to Wednesday. They don't work on Fridays.'

Our stomach drops, but Eliza doesn't seem concerned. She smiles warmly, apologising for the mix-up and, after a brief conversation, smoothly arranges for us to visit a different class instead.

The school feels strangely quiet. There are no signs of the children beyond the sound of soft, cheerful singing coming faintly from a distant classroom. *'If you're happy and you know it, stomp your feet.'*

We're anxious and can't concentrate properly. The woman at the office mistakes our obvious nervousness for fear of teaching. 'You'll be fine,' she says, filling the kettle and opening a biscuit tin. 'We're a good-natured bunch. You'll do well here. I can feel it. I'm Marnie, by the way. Is it tea or coffee to begin the day?'

Eliza calls Nathan to let him know we've arrived safely. 'We're just signing in,' she tells him. She passes the phone to Marnie. 'Sorry,' she says quietly. 'It's Laurie-Amelia's Support Worker. He just wants to confirm their whereabouts.'

Marnie takes the phone with a reassuring smile. We watch tensely as she cradles it between her shoulder and cheek as she pours boiling water over the tea bags. 'Yes, yes,' she says. 'A little trepidatious but that's to be expected. Don't worry, we'll look after them.'

We can't finish our tea, but we manage a biscuit. It's dry and sticks to the roof of our mouth, making speaking difficult. We nod or shake our head when Marnie asks us a question.

'You needn't be shy around me, pet,' she says. 'I'm not one to judge or criticise. I'm in awe of all of you Combines. I really am.' She smiles warmly. 'Let's get going, shall we?'

We leave Eliza at the front office. She settles into an armchair by the window, unfolding a newspaper and smoothing out its creases. 'Take your time,' she says. 'I'm in no rush to get back.'

We smile and nod, offering a small smile. She turns her attention to the paper.

Marnie leads us down a quiet corridor to a classroom at the back of the school, beyond the boundary of the privet hedge. Through the windows, a lush green field slopes away into the distance. We imagine it at playtime, full of laughter and chatter, children racing each other, sprinting up and down the hill, their energy uncontainable. Teachers supervising, advising the children to not run so fast. *It's wet*, they say, *you might slip and hurt yourself.*

'Laurie-Amelia, meet Teacher Pilkington,' Marnie says. 'They're happy to have you join their class this morning. You enjoy yourself. If you need me, I'll be in the office. I'm happy to lend an ear whenever required.' She winks before leaving the classroom.

'It's lovely to meet you, Laurie-Amelia. I'm Philippa-Thomas. Teacher Pilkington to the children. And to Marnie, apparently.' They smile. A calm, gentle Combine, beanpole thin, with long limbs and receding hair. The children clearly adore them; their little hands shoot up with every question Teacher Pilkington asks.

They're sweet children. All ten in the class have a Host age of six, but it's easy to spot the ones who have merged with older Transfers. They tell us stories of their past lives.

'I jumped out of a plane once,' a little Combine called Erica-Alice says as they colour in, their pink crayon straying well beyond the lines. 'With a golden parachute. I did it when I was in Australia. Did you know there are kangaroos in Australia? They carry their babies in a pouch in their tummy and they bounce like this.' Erica-Alice abandons their colouring and starts hopping around the classroom.

The children are adorably innocent. It's disconcerting whenever we catch sight of their mandala tattoos peeking out from under their collars. There's a great deal of laughter and play, and slowly, we find ourselves relaxing. For a moment, we forget this is only a tour, that we have no real intention of taking the role.

Perhaps we should go back into teaching when we leave here. What do you think? I'm really enjoying myself, are you?

Nothing.

'Come and see my pine-cone family, Assistant Anderson.' We're pulled by the hand to Polly-Connor's table. They have a mop of chestnut hair and, when they smile, we notice they're missing one of their front teeth.

On the table, a row of pine cones is neatly arranged by size. 'This is the daddy pine cone,' they explain, pointing at the largest. 'And this is the mummy. And these are all of their babies. There are too many babies so they're merging. Then they can have more money for holidays.' They begin flicking the smallest pine cones onto the floor, one by one. 'Now there are only two babies.' They grin, proudly showing off their gap-toothed smile. 'That's better because of the embiro-ment.'

We smile faintly, running a hand over their unruly hair. 'How old was Polly?'

'A baby,' they say happily.

We nod. It would be the easier choice.

A loud cry erupts from the corner of the room. A little Combine screams, distraught as another takes the train they were playing with. Teacher Pilkington is distracted, hurrying over to mediate.

We seize the opportunity.

We slip out of the room and hurry down the corridor, its fluorescent lights casting a harsh, sterile glow on the pale walls. The echoes of children's chatter and laughter fade behind us.

At the end of the corridor, we find the door Eliza told us about, painted a dull grey, with a push-bar for easy exit. Glancing around to ensure no one is watching, we press down on the bar. It makes a satisfying click, and the door swings open, letting in a rush of crisp, fresh air.

We step outside and walk quickly away from the building, our head lowered. We pass the school gardener, crouched over an ancient lawnmower. He spots us and smiles.

'I'm always tinkering with her, keeping her going,' he says. 'She was a real beauty in her day. They keep offering me a new one, but I'm too old for that. We get along well enough, don't we.' He pats the mower affectionately, like it's an old dog.

We smile politely, murmuring a vague response before strolling away, as if we have all the time in the world. The moment we're out of his sight, we break into a run. By the time we reach the path lined with red-brick houses, we're sprinting.

It takes us less than five minutes to reach Benjamin-Annie's house. We pause at the gate, catching our breath, glancing over our shoulder, scanning for any sign of being followed.

We hurry through the front garden, our breath shallow and quick, and slip round to the back of the house.

At the first window, we crouch low, keeping out of sight as we peer inside. Angela is in the kitchen, singing along to the radio while she dices potatoes, the thud of her knife rhythmic against the chopping board.

There's no sign of Benjamin-Annie.

We move to the next window. The curtains are drawn, but a narrow gap offers just enough space for us to catch a glimpse inside. Holding our breath, we lean closer, straining to see what lies behind the curtains.

It's the nursery.

Benjamin-Annie sits slumped in a rocking chair, their head lolling to one side. They're in pyjamas, their hair unkempt, their bright-red curls spiralling in unruly tangles.

We gently tap on the window, but there's no response. They don't even flinch.

We scan the room, searching for Teddy. The crib is tucked just out of view.

But then we spot him – small and still, fast asleep in Benjamin-Annie's lap.

We tap again, louder this time, hoping to stir some reaction. The only answer is the low hum of white noise from a machine and the slow creak of the rocking chair.

They remain motionless.

We knock harder, the window frame rattling.

What's wrong with them? Why aren't they moving?

They seem more than just asleep, as if they've slipped into a state where no amount of noise could rouse them. An uneasy weight settles in the pit of our stomach.

Angela enters the nursery, a blanket draped over her arm. We quickly duck below the window, pressing ourselves against the wall, our heart pounding. We grip the window ledge and slowly inch upwards, peering cautiously over the edge as Angela moves towards Benjamin-Annie.

She picks up Teddy with one hand, tucks him neatly under her arm, then drapes the blanket across Benjamin-Annie's lap. Gently, she places Teddy back on their lap, nestling him against their chest. He remains quiet, completely still.

'There, there,' Angela mutters, her voice soft as she strokes Benjamin-Annie's forehead.

We hold our breath, waiting for something. Anything. A flicker of movement from Benjamin-Annie, another word from Angela, a cry from Teddy.

Nothing.

We inch closer, craning our neck to get a better look at Teddy. His skin is so smooth it looks almost artificial. His blue eyes stare ahead, unblinking, fixed in a vacant gaze. His face is expressionless, unnervingly still.

And we realise.

It's not Teddy. It's a doll.

We turn cold, our breath catching in our throat. We clutch the windowsill, our hands trembling, and scan the room. *Where is he? Where's Teddy?*

Then we hear it – a voice.

Faint but unmistakable, coming from somewhere behind the drawn curtains.

'I remember when I was a kid and I'd wait all week to go to the corner shop…'

We edge forward, straining to catch the rest.

'…I'd save up. I got ten pence a day for making my bed. Then on Sunday, I'd spend it all. I'd pick the penny sweets, so I could get the most. Cola bottles were my favourite…'

We let go of the windowsill. The voice doesn't belong to Annie or Angela.

It's a man's voice, low and familiar.

Ben.

'…I'd like to start the tradition with my child when they're old enough. We could ride our bikes to the corner shop on a Sunday. I'll get the paper, and my child can get the sweets…' The voice fades, and is replaced by the familiar hiss of white noise. It rises and falls like the sea.

We stagger backwards.

The white noise.

There, Nathan always said, to help us relax.

He was so insistent, relentless. 'It's vital you get enough sleep,' he'd say. 'Without it you won't fully align.'

Benjamin-Annie sits motionless, sedated, their mind saturated by Ben's voice, his words seeping into their dreams, their subconscious.

If that's happening to them, then who's to say…

A quiet voice behind us breaks through our thoughts, making us jump.

'I'm so sorry, Amelia. I didn't know how to tell you.'

We freeze, every muscle rigid.

'What did you call me?'

Eliza whispers, her voice barely audible, as if she's afraid of the word.

'Amelia.'

The drugs, regular at first, then given less often, until eventually we only took them before bed, before naps, before drifting off into unconsciousness.

All those dreams – if they were dreams – never from Amelia's perspective. Never her memories. Only Laurie's. Always Laurie's.

So real, so vivid.

And as the pills were reduced, the dreams became harder to reach. We'd jolt awake, certain we'd heard a voice.

An intruder.

Not an intruder after all, but a recording.

Whenever we slept, Nathan would switch on the white noise. 'It helps you,' he'd say. 'You need it to get a good night's sleep.'

We look again at Benjamin-Annie, lifeless in their rocking chair.

'Look, Laurie-Amelia,' Nathan would say, his voice brimming with pride as he showed us our brilliant sleep score. Night after night. Always so pleased. Always so proud. 'You're doing wonderfully. Keep this up, and you'll have no trouble at all in aligning.'

Our sleep score, tracked. Recorded.

The watch...

We look at our wrist.

Then at Eliza.

She's sitting beneath the window, her face a waterlogged sponge. 'The watch tracks your sleep patterns,' she whispers. 'It's linked to the white-noise machine. The machine plays recordings – like the one of Ben – but only when you're in a deep sleep. The white noise drowns them out otherwise.'

All those nights we woke to the hissing, like escaping gas. Never a voice, even when we were sure someone had spoken.

'Show me.'

Eliza closes her eyes, shaking her head, refusing to meet our gaze.

'Show me the recordings I've been hearing.'

'I can't.'

'Show me, or I'll scream,' we threaten, our voice wavering. 'I'll say you've told me everything. That you brought me here. I'll tell them I saw you with Albie, that you're working with him, with the anti—'

'Amelia—'

We open our mouth to scream, but she clamps her hand over it, her touch cold and trembling. A flicker of memory surfaces. Rough hands, muffled cries.

'Okay,' she whispers, her voice shaky. 'Okay. But I need your watch.'

We extend our wrist, watching as she activates a screen we've never seen before, her hands unsteady as she enters a four-digit code.

We watch nervously as she continues to fiddle with our watch. She could be doing anything, sending out a distress signal, calling for help. *Laurie-Amelia is on the loose. At Benjamin-Annie's house. Send backup.*

Finally, the watch beeps. Eliza exhales, her relief audible. 'I've got to change the settings to make it seem as though you're in a deep sleep,' she mutters, her grip tight on our wrist. She continues pressing buttons, then abruptly releases her hand.

The white noise from the nursery cuts off.

In its place, a voice begins to play through the machine.

'Oh no, I'm blind as a bat without my contact lenses,' it says, light-hearted and cheerful.

It's Mum. Me. Us.

She sounds almost giddy, like she's on the verge of laughter. 'For years, I had to wear glasses. Amelia was terrified of eyes – even her own. It drove Mitchell mad. She couldn't stand it when I put in my contact lenses. It always made her squirm to see my fingertip so close to my eye...'

What the fuck.

We pull ourselves up and peer back through the gap in the curtains.

Benjamin-Annie's head is still drooping, their arm dangling limply at their side.

'You remind me of someone from my childhood, Nathan,' Mum's voice continues. 'Walter Green was his name. He lived opposite in a small bungalow. He put me up whenever I wasn't able to go home. He never asked questions, at least not to me. He just let me sit with him, playing board games until it was time for bed. I got to be very good at draughts... Sometimes he took me to school the next morning. I always had cornflakes for breakfast with milk straight from the fridge. I love cold milk with cornflakes...'

A pause.

Then another voice comes through, deep and unmistakable. Nathan.

'Did he ever help, Laurie?'

We know what's coming. Word for word. The answer is burned into our memory. We mouth along with it, tears blurring our vision until Benjamin-Annie is no longer visible through the window. 'He called the police once. My mother hated him for doing that, but I never did. I liked knowing he was there, looking out for us.'

Eliza presses a button on our watch, and the white noise floods back in, swallowing up the voices.

The nursery feels colder. Emptier. Benjamin-Annie remains slumped in the rocking chair, their posture lifeless.

We clutch the windowsill, the recordings pressing down, rooting us to the spot.

'Are you okay, Amelia? Shall I keep going?'

Can you handle hearing more?

We wait, straining for an answer, but nothing comes.

We give a slow nod.

Mum's voice fills the room again, her words edged with pain.

'I remember one time we'd been to the park. Or maybe it was the woods. Somewhere muddy. Tony started shouting as soon as we walked through the door… He reached for me before I was able to take my shoes off. I dodged him, ran upstairs and traipsed mud all over their room. He hit my mother for that. He smacked her. He split her lip right open. I sat upstairs and listened from their bedroom, rubbing my bare feet against the carpet as she received the punishment that was intended for me.'

There's a sniff. A pause.

'Do you know that he believed himself to be a good person? He honestly thought he had morals. He took us to church every Sunday. And he prayed every night. He tried to preach to us, to tell us what it meant to be a good person. In my experience, the people who spend their time preaching about loving and being kind to others are often the cruellest individuals. The good people, the people who would never think to do otherwise, don't feel kindness is something that needs to be taught. It's the people who preach about being a good person. They're the worst ones out there.'

The white noise rolls back in.

We're thrown back to the church on the day of our Passing. The tension. The nausea pooling in our stomach. The weight of his hand on our leg, the unspoken threat it carried.

The hum fades, giving way to Mum's voice.

'The day Amelia was born, I felt delirious with love. That first moment, when our bodies touched, skin on skin, both of us crying. Amelia terrified of the bright new world, me trembling with love. I can still feel it, how that love poured into my life like a flood, unstoppable and overwhelming. But it was so difficult to relax. After losing Harrison... I took no risks. I'd spend the nights watching her, guarding her as she slept. I had this need to protect her from everything. Even when Mitchell would hold her, I couldn't properly relax. The only time I felt I could breathe easily was when she was in my arms. It was like caring for my mother all over again.'

'Tell me about how your mother died, Laurie. Talk me through it. I know you said she took her own life. How exactly? It's important you become comfortable speaking about these things. It's the only way the memories won't overwhelm Amelia when you merge...'

'I got home from a date... I found her in the bathtub. She was lying there... The water was almost black with blood...'

We double over, retching violently, spitting bitter liquid that scalds our throat.

The image is seared into our mind – the red water, her lifeless body, the quiet, suffocating horror.

We knew this. It was always there, buried in our thoughts, haunting our dreams. But we never confronted it. Never spoke about it when we had the chance, before the voices in our head fell silent. We could have opened up. Could have faced it together, confronted the nightmares as one.

But we were too scared. Too proud. Too afraid to fully expose the raw, broken parts of ourselves.

So we kept it buried.

'I can still see it, clear as day. Her arm was hanging limply over the edge. There was blood pooling on the tiles...'

Why didn't you tell me?

The question screams through our mind. *Did you think I couldn't handle it?*

Answer me, for fuck's sake. Why did you keep this from me? Were you trying to protect me? Shield me from your pain?

Tears fall, hot and bitter, mingling with the guilt tightening our chest.

We straighten, wiping our mouth with the back of our hand. *How could I have missed it? How could I have been so blind to your silent struggle?*

'I stayed there for hours,' Mum's voice continues, 'watching the drip, drip of her blood. It was murder, you know, not suicide. She might have finally taken her own life, but it's only because she was so terrified. He killed her. If it wasn't for him, she'd have lived. She'd have met Mitchell and Amelia.'

We're not sure whether the crying is coming from us or the machine, not until the white noise resumes, and the sobbing stops.

We turn to Eliza. 'Everything coming from these recordings... that was what we spoke about...'

Eliza nods.

'And what we saw in our dreams...'

A bitter taste stings the back of our throat as we swallow. Eliza's face has gone pale. She reaches out for our hand, but we step back.

'Amelia...'

'These recordings have been playing while we've been asleep?'

She nods.

Our finger hovers above the button Eliza's been pressing to get the recordings to play. A part of us screams to run, to get as far from this machine as physically possible.

But the other part of us needs to know.

How can we understand what's been fed to us, and what's real, if we don't listen?

With a deep breath, we close our eyes. And then we press the button.

'Amelia relies on being in control.' Mum's voice is calm. 'It's why we're doing this. My Alzheimer's isn't something she can control unless we merge, unless she literally takes over. I always find it remarkable how different we are in that respect. Not knowing what's coming doesn't worry me. She takes after her father. Mitchell needed to know exactly what was happening too. Not in an overbearing way. I once worked with a woman who kept her class timetable hidden so that the poor children never knew what to expect. It made one little boy so unbearably anxious that he stopped coming to school altogether. She needed the power. Amelia's not like that. She just wants to be sure everything is going to be okay. It *is* going to be okay, isn't it?'

The recordings continue, an endless stream of relentless, often mundane, conversation. We sit with our back to the wall, eyes closed, trying to remain composed.

There's nothing new, nothing we haven't already discussed during head-talk or experienced in a dream. Nothing we couldn't recite by heart.

It isn't the content of the recordings that twists our stomach. It's the realisation that we've been manipulated, that our minds – our memories – have been infiltrated without our knowledge.

Every word, every detail, meticulously placed.

And all this time, we thought we were dreaming.

Remembering.

Nathan's voice filters through the machine now, smooth and matter-of-fact. 'You said it was extremely important, Laurie. I need to document anything of major importance. You know that.'

'Fine, look, I'm sure I've asked this countless times before but, Nathan, I need to know. Will I be able to retain memories of events that Amelia didn't experience? I understand she'll be able to help me recall moments she has been privy to. But what about the conversations she's not around for? Important ones that I need to remember.'

'We can't be certain she'll have access to those, of course, but the hope is that your memories will restore, including the ones that are yours and yours alone.'

'It's vital that I remember this. If I don't... Well, Amelia and I... We'll struggle tremendously.'

'May I ask what it is?'

There's a pause. The faint sound of paper being unfolded.

'Silly sod?'

'I know it seems stupid. But I need to remember it.'

'I'm not following, Laurie.'

A long silence follows.

We will the conversation to end, hoping Mum will leave it there. Hoping this won't go any further.

But her voice returns.

'Mary's given me a codeword. She wants proof, following our Merge, that I'm still there. If I forget it, then I won't be able to prove that it's worked, will I? But I can't tell Amelia the codeword, can't ask her to remember it for me, otherwise that defeats the purpose. I need to call Mary a silly sod when she asks for proof that I'm there. I need to remember *silly sod*.'

We close our eyes, our body convulsing with sobs.

Eliza wraps her arms round us, holding us tightly as we tremble uncontrollably.

'I need to call Mary a silly sod when she asks for proof that I'm there. I need to remember *silly sod*. I need to call Mary a silly sod when she asks for proof that I'm there. I need to remember *silly sod*. I need to call Mary a silly sod when she asks for proof that I'm there. I need to remember *silly sod*.'

The sentence loops endlessly, relentlessly, until we can't take it anymore. We press the button, silencing the voice.

'Amelia,' Eliza whispers softly. 'We have to get you back to the apartment. We've been gone far too long, and Nathan—'

We look around The Enclave.

Home to children.

Children.

Toddlers learning to read and write. Polly-Connor flicking the pine cones off the table. Erica-Alice bouncing around the classroom. They've been taken from their family. Put forward for the Merge *by* their family. Forced to live apart from their parents, from their siblings.

Children, all indelibly marked with the symbol of Combines.

Children.

Without a say, without a choice. Too young to decide their own fate.

Lara.

We think of Lara-Jay, that walk when they finally spoke, their cheek pressed against the gravel: *I can't hear her. Why can't I hear her?*

We stand, our legs trembling, and look in at Benjamin-Annie. Out cold.

The drugs. Stashed in the teddy bears. Never swallowed.

'Lara-Jay never took the pills,' we whisper.

Eliza nods, her expression heavy. 'They were terrified of becoming addicted to Narcoproxitin. It isn't a dangerous drug, Amelia. We wouldn't prescribe it if it was. But they were so scared. So, they didn't take it. I thought…' She swallows, her voice faltering. 'Jay regularly spoke of his fear of being medicated. I thought I'd put his mind at ease, that I'd convinced him Lara's addictive tendencies wouldn't be a problem with the prescription drugs, that I'd be monitoring them closely enough to ensure there was never an issue. But he clearly didn't believe me. So he... Well, you know as well as I do.'

'What do the drugs do?' we whisper.

Eliza looks through the window at Benjamin-Annie, her eyes clouded with guilt. 'It's like a sleeping pill, but it does more than just put you to sleep. It relaxes your mental inhibitions and opens your consciousness, making your mind highly receptive to suggestions when sedated, a sort of medicated hypnotic state. That's how the recordings work, they infiltrate your thoughts. If you don't take the pills, the suggestions can't take hold. That's why Lara-Jay remained unaffected. They never ingested the pills.'

'So the whole time they were here in The Village...'

'I doubt they experienced any head-talk.' She sniffs, her voice cracking slightly. 'I didn't know about any of this, Amelia. I promise. I would never have... It was only after Lara-Jay died and we found their medication. It was you, Amelia. You opened my eyes. You showed me something was wrong. I started talking to anti-Mergers, people I'd always believed to be crazy. I needed to see if I had them wrong too, if they had answers I couldn't find anywhere else. That's when I met Albie. He's been critical in helping me piece this together, Amelia. He hasn't rested. It was Albie who first suggested that the white noise might be part of the problem.'

We think of Lara-Jay's cough, the way their slow, heavy movements seemed weighed down by grief.

'And Benjamin-Annie?' we ask. 'Why did they say Combine had taken Ben? Why couldn't they hear him?'

'Annie was pregnant, Amelia. They couldn't risk drugging her as heavily. They couldn't risk harming the baby, but that meant she was more lucid, less susceptible to merging. It's why we kept her apart from you, even after Teddy was born. I wanted to reunite you. I really, really did. So did Nathan. He was just waiting until he was told she was healthy.'

We stare at Eliza. 'She?'

'Annie.'

Not Ben. Not both. Just... Annie.

'Where's Mum?' we whisper, barely able to form the words. 'If she's not here, then where is she?'

Eliza looks at us. 'I'm so sorry, Amelia.'

Her lips keep moving, but we—

No.

There is no we.

It's just... me.

Just me. Alone.

I shake my head, the denial rising like bile. 'It doesn't make sense. Mum can't be... My dementia. It's here. It's never gone. I've never been cured, Eliza.'

'You've never had dementia, Amelia,' she says softly.

'But all those blanks... I've forgotten so much... I...'

'You believe you have dementia, so, naturally, every small thing that slips your mind feels significant. It feels like the disease. But all Combines – all *humans* – forget things, Amelia. Those weeks leading up to your Merge weren't forgotten. They were taken from you. If you really think about it, what have you forgotten since being in The Village? In all the time we've spent together, you've never once forgotten my name. Your mum used to forget me from one session to the next.'

The truth crashes down with brutal clarity.

There is no 'we'. There never was.

It's always been just me, clinging to a delusion that I wasn't in this alone. But she's gone. Mum is gone.

Buried by the very people who took her. The ones who decided she was expendable, who rendered her life meaningless in their relentless pursuit of progress.

Grief wells up, a churning, stabbing pain in my chest, so fierce it's hard to breathe.

Gone.

Mum, who held me when I was scared, who whispered stories in the dark to chase away my nightmares after Dad died, even as she drowned in her own grief. Mum, who laughed with me in the kitchen, flour dusting her cheeks as we baked biscuits, always burnt or raw, but it never mattered. Mum, who sacrificed everything for me, only to be sacrificed by them.

The agony is relentless, every memory cutting deeper. She was my everything, my anchor, my compass. And they took her. Killed her.

I think of her notebook, how often she pulled me aside, her voice urgent as she shared her fears. The lists she'd written of everything that seemed wrong about the Merge. The things that didn't add up. The things that scared her.

She knew.

She knew the Merge wasn't what it seemed. And I forced her into it.

'Eliza,' I whisper. 'Did we... Did we decide to merge? Or... were we...'

Eliza's eyes meet mine, and the answer is already there. 'It was too late to back out,' she says quietly. 'You were pushed into it. It wasn't your choice. I'm so sorry, Amelia.'

Her words settle over me like a heavy fog.

Slowly, a realisation begins to unfold. 'Mary,' I whisper, her name a fragile breath on my lips.

'What?'

'Nathan said she was going to—' My voice catches, breaking like brittle glass. 'Oh my god.' I stagger backwards, my body weakening as the truth crashes into me. Mary witnessed a Combine take their own life, and she was killed for it. Silenced.

I cover my mouth, bile rising. 'Does Albie know what's happening? Did you tell him?'

'I couldn't, Amelia. They'd kill me. I did what I could. I got him into the party, and I told him I'd get you out. I—'

'Nathan…'

Her expression shifts, her panic immediate. 'He doesn't know. None of the Support Workers know what's—'

Her eyes widen, and the little colour left in her face drains away.

Strong hands grip my shoulders.

'Get off!' Eliza cries, lunging towards me to yank them away, but a heavy blow sends her crashing to the ground.

A scream. Then silence.

The silence terrifies me.

I twist, just in time to see the flash of a syringe.

'No.' The word spills from me, frantic, raw. I shake my head, thrashing against the iron grip holding me in place. 'No, please, Nathan. Don't—'

My vision is blurred. Hazy. Like looking through smeared glass.

I try to lift my head. Slowly, slowly. It takes so much effort. Too much. My head slumps again, and I have to lift my right hand with my left. Drag it up. Move it like a puppet.

I stare at the screen. Something's playing. An image of Noah-Lucas. Beside them, Callie smiles. Trees hung with bunting. Bright flags. They sway. The voice coming from the TV is muffled. I can't make out all the words. Only catch snippets.

...*courageous soul... nurturing walls of The Village... remarkable transformation...*

'Isn't this exciting, Laurie-Amelia.' A clink behind me. Porcelain. The chime of a spoon. Tea being made. The man sounds calm. Happy. He laughs, as if we're sharing a joke. 'Don't feel bad. This will be you before you know it.'

I squint at the screen. There's a crowd now. Someone's hugging Noah-Lucas. They turn their face to the camera. Squinting. Trying to see. Ellie.

Ellie.

They kiss. The crowd cheers.

There's a knock on the door.

'That'll be them, just in time.' The man moves past me, out of the lounge. Then back. He's brought two women with him. One pushes a wheelchair. The other's sitting in it, slumped forward.

The man smiles. His teeth gleam, unnaturally white. Too white. 'Look who's here to see you,' he says.

I stare at the wheelchair. The person in it. Small. Hunched. Curled in on herself. Tangled hair covering her face.

'Hello, Laurie-Amelia.' Angela's voice. Too bright. Too sweet. 'We thought it would be fun to watch Noah-Lucas's departing statement with you. Mr Brightwell mentioned you've been asking after Benjamin-Annie, and I know they'll be delighted to be in your company.'

'Isn't that kind, Laurie-Amelia?' Brightwell's voice – cheerful, almost sing-song. 'It's been a while since you two spent time together.'

I lift my hand. Reaching for Benjamin-Annie. Fingers trembling.

A baby, Amelia. Look. A baby.

Angela crouches in front of Benjamin-Annie. She speaks slowly. Gentle. Careful. 'I'm going to take Teddy from you now. Just for a moment, just until you're sitting comfortably on the sofa with Laurie-Amelia. Then I'll hand him back, okay?'

Benjamin-Annie stares. Doesn't move.

Angela lifts Teddy from their arms. Places him beside me on the sofa, wrapped tight in a green blanket. I stare. 'Quiet,' I say. Words feel thick. Strange in my mouth. 'Nice and quiet.'

Brightwell nods, strokes Teddy's tiny head. Silky hair. Soft. 'Yes, Laurie-Amelia. Teddy is a good little boy. He's so extraordinarily calm. Not like me when I was that age. I bawled incessantly, so I'm told.'

Benjamin-Annie smiles. They reach for Teddy. Angela hands him back, places him carefully in their arms. Benjamin-Annie holds him close. Kisses his head.

'Small,' I whisper. 'Tiny baby.'

Angela sits between me and Benjamin-Annie. Blocks me. Brightwell settles back in his armchair. His cup is painted with daisies. He sips. Sips and watches.

'Isn't this nice?' he says.

...celebration of survival... triumphant return to society... a story of rebirth, of strength and extraordinary potential...

The words coming from the TV blur, blend. Merging with

the recording playing from the speaker in the corner. Over and over. Mum's voice.

I never told anyone I was pregnant. Not even your father. It was a terrible secret. All I wanted was to scream the truth, to tell everyone about the miracle growing inside of me. But I was too scared. I didn't want to jinx it...

Angela's voice. 'I wonder if Eliza and Nathan are watching Noah-Lucas's speech. Or Eliza-James and Nathan-Owen, should I say. They must have completed their Merges by now.' She tilts her head thoughtfully. 'I hope Noah-Lucas's departure is being broadcast in their Villages.'

'Oh, it will be,' Brightwell says. 'The whole world will be tuning in.'

On the screen: Noah-Lucas. Speaking. Cheeks pink. Fringe fluttering. I want to tell Brightwell: *Turn up the volume.* Or: *Turn off the recording.* It's too much. I can't follow.

...Combine have given me a future... the past five years... no longer defined by my illness...

Noah-Lucas's eyes shine. So close to crying.

I think of Brightwell's speech earlier. So proud of Noah-Lucas. So good. They've done so well. Deserved this more than I ever could. Never doubted the Merge's potential. Always trusted. Always listened.

...valuable lessons... strength... boundless capacity for change... can't thank you enough... happier than I've ever been...

Brightwell's smile stretches wider, wider. Looks painful. Like his face might tear open.

Benjamin-Annie doesn't watch the screen. They stare only at Teddy. Only at their son.

The speech continues.

...a life-saving decision... transformative... thank the founders, scientists, Support Workers...

'Can I hold? Please?'

Benjamin-Annie looks up. Their eyes meet mine. Slowly, they nod. Angela smiles. Takes Teddy from Benjamin-Annie. Places him in my arms. He's light. So light.

Then I remember.

I look down. His plastic face. Doll-limbs.

I sit perfectly still. Hold him like he's real. Like he might wake.

...paved the way for a future free of cancer... seemingly insurmountable challenges... rewrite the narrative of our lives... full of new adventures...

Noah-Lucas's speech ends. The cheers, loud. So loud.

Benjamin-Annie stares. Anxious. Desperate. Reaches for Teddy.

'What on earth?' Angela shifts beside us. Uneasy.

The TV chants. A familiar sound.

I lift my head. Squint at the screen. Noah-Lucas is gone. Replaced.

A crowd. Raised placards. Shaky camera.

Protestors. All ages.

An old woman. Face set, determined, holding a sign. A young man, wild hair, middle finger to the lens. A mother clutching her child, shielding their face.

Smoke bomb. Yellow fog. Screams.

Teenage girls run, blind. Eyes wide. Two men, hands tight on a friend's arm. Dragging him from the cloud. He collapses. Coughing. Choking.

In the chaos, someone charges at the camera.

I gasp.

Albie.

Sweat-soaked. Eyes wide, wild. Scanning, searching. He yells, his words lost, drowned.

Camera jerks, swings.

A woman, blood streaming, pulled to safety. A man, placard raised like a weapon. Rage. Fear. Everywhere.

More protestors. More chaos. Human barricade.

A young couple, arms locked, shouting together. A teen with a bandana hurls a canister back. An older man, hair matted, fist high, bellowing.

Chanting. Louder. Clearer.

Not just the TV.

Outside. Here. In The Village.

Their message is clear.

Unstoppable.

Merge is murder.

Angela's hand on my shoulder. Firm. Grounding. 'Don't worry. This won't last long. Security will handle it.'

Brightwell sets his cup down. Looks to the window.

On the screen, Albie again. Running. His face flashes between smoke and chaos. Swinging placards and flailing arms.

He's close, so close.

I reach for him.

'Laurie-Amelia?' Angela's voice. Sharper now. Her fingers tight on my shoulder. 'Why don't we focus on Teddy? He's feeling a little... overwhelmed.'

I glance at the doll. Painted eyes. My hands tremble. I tighten my grip.

Outside, a crash. Glass shatters. A scream.

Angela stands. She and Brightwell rush to the window.

My head jerks. Watches. Smoke curls past the edges of the frame.

Benjamin-Annie's hand on mine.

Their eyes wide, pleading. Fixed on the doll in my arms.

Teddy. Their baby.

Another crash. Another scream.

Benjamin-Annie's lips move. Silent. Mouthing a single word: *Please.*

The Support Workers – still by the window. Faces close to the glass.

Watching.

It's now.

My chance.

Fight through the fog. One final push.

I nod.

Okay.

Acknowledgements

There are rare, extraordinary people who not only recognise potential in others but nurture it, challenge it, and ensure it never goes unnoticed. In my life, that person is Gary Mepsted.

When I signed up for a six-week writing course in 2017, I had no idea that my tutor, Gary, would become one of my dearest friends and the reason this book exists. More than anyone, I owe him my deepest thanks, not only for helping this novel find its way into the world but for discovering the writer in me. Gary, your generosity with your time, your endless patience with my limited spatial awareness, and the countless hours you've spent guiding me have been a gift beyond measure. Thank you for making me speak up when I was terrified to share my work, for teaching me to persevere through doubt, and for reminding me, always, that the writing itself is what truly matters. Without you, I doubt I'd ever have finished a first draft. For that – and for all the laughter along the way – I am forever grateful.

Mum and Dad. Your unwavering love and support have given me the courage to chase this dream, and I could not be more grateful. How lucky I am to have you. Thank you for everything, including your constant (and wildly inaccurate) claims of spotting yourselves in my characters. I promise, if I ever write you in, you'll know!

My sister, Emma. Growing up watching you devour novel after novel made literature feel exciting, a gift that shaped both my childhood and my future. Your generous advice, encouragement and belief in me have been a constant source of strength. Thank you.

My irreplaceable friends and chosen family, Sheryl Jared and Natasha Dean. Thank you for celebrating every milestone, no matter how small. That screaming phone call when I got the book deal and the celebrations that followed meant everything to me. I am so lucky to have you both in my corner. Tasha, thank you for being my biggest cheerleader and the first to read every draft with such enthusiasm and care. Sometimes, knowing that just one person enjoys your work is enough to make years of trying feel worthwhile. I'm sorry for making you cry on a plane.

To all my wonderful writing friends who have been there for the highs and lows – most notably Silvia Saunders, Liz Breen, Amy Abdelnoor, Lucy Mepsted and Jim Harris – your support and advice have shaped this novel in more ways than you realise. Your honesty, encouragement and kindness have enriched both my writing and my life. Thank you for always being there to turn to.

My incredible agent, Liv Maidment. Your brilliance, creativity and infinite support have shaped this novel into what it is today. I am endlessly grateful that you took a chance on me and my manuscript, and for your guidance and dedication every step of the way. To the entire team at Madeleine Milburn, thank you for the incredible work that happens behind the scenes.

My hugely talented editors, Jessica Vestuto, Jenny Parrott and Wayne Brookes. Your meticulous attention, insight and enthusiasm have been truly transformative. I'm endlessly grateful to have such gifted and generous minds guiding my work. I still can't believe my luck. And to everyone at Mariner and Oneworld, thank you for taking a chance on this book and for your dedication to bringing it to life.

Finally, to Jim. Like with everything in life, you made writing this book an adventure. Thank you for the brainstorming sessions, for covering the walls of our flat in sticky notes, and for talking about these characters as if they were part of our lives. Thank you for putting up with me writing on every holiday, for tolerating my 4 a.m. writing sessions, and for always knowing exactly what to say when I doubted myself. Your patience, love and unwavering support mean more to me than words can express. You always insist you haven't done anything, but, honestly, I couldn't have done this without you. Your love is, and always will be, the greatest gift of all.